Deinstitutionalization and People with Intellectual Disabilities

by the same authors

Women With Intellectual Disabilities
Finding a Place in the World
Edited by Rannveig Traustadóttir and Kelley Johnson
ISBN 1 85302 846 0

Inclusive Research with People with Learning Disabilities
Past, Present and Futures
Jan Walmsley and Kelley Johnson
ISBN 1 84310 061 4

of related interest

Working with People with Learning Disabilities
Theory and Practice
David Thomas and Honor Woods
ISBN 1 85302 973 4

Transition and Change in the Lives of People with Intellectual Disabilities
Edited by David May
Research Highlights in Social Work 38
ISBN 1 85302 863 0

Person Centred Planning and Care Management with People with Learning Disabilities
Edited by Paul Cambridge and Steven Carnaby
ISBN 1 84310 131 9

Guide to Mental Health for Families and Carers of People with Intellectual Disabilities
Geraldine Holt, Anastasia Gratsa, Nick Bouras, Teresa Joyce, Mary Jane Spiller and Steve Hardy
ISBN 1 84310 277 3

Quality of Life and Disability
An Approach for Community Practitioners
Ivan Brown and Roy I. Brown
Foreword by Ann and Rud Turnbull
ISBN 1 84310 005 3

Advocacy and Learning Disability
Edited by Barry Gray and Robin Jackson
ISBN 1 85302 942 4

Deinstitutionalization and People with Intellectual Disabilities

In and Out of Institutions

Edited by

Kelley Johnson and Rannveig Traustadóttir

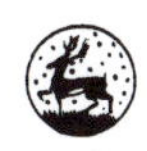

Jessica Kingsley Publishers
London and Philadelphia

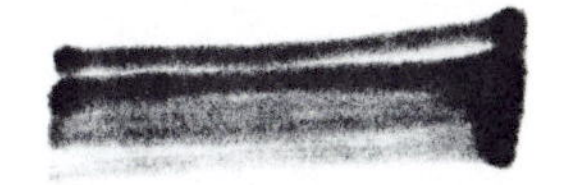

First published in 2005
by Jessica Kingsley Publishers
116 Pentonville Road
London N1 9JB, UK
and
400 Market Street, Suite 400
Philadelphia, PA 19106, USA

www.jkp.com

Library of Congress Cataloging in Publication Data

Deinstitutionalization and people with intellectual disabilities : in and out of institutions / edited by Kelley Johnson and Rannveig Traustadóttir.— 1st American paperback ed.

p. cm.

Includes bibliographical references and index.

ISBN-13: 978-1-84310-101-7 (pbk. : alk. paper)

ISBN-10: 1-84310-101-7 (pbk. : alk. paper) 1. People with mental disabilities—Deinstitutionalization—Cross-cultural studies. 2. Mental retardation facilities. I. Johnson, Kelley, 1947- II. Rannveig Traustadóttir, 1950-

HV3004.D42 2005

362.2'2—dc22

2005011552

British Library Cataloguing in Publication Data

A CIP catalogue record for this book is available from the British Library

ISBN-13: 978 1 84310 101 7
ISBN-10: 1 84310 101 7

Printed and Bound in Great Britain by
Athenaeum Press, Gateshead, Tyne and Wear

This book is written in loving memory of
Tom Allen 1912–1991
and dedicated to our children Rúna and Sam

Contents

Acknowledgements

This book has been many years in the making and its roots reach far into our pasts. Along the way numerous people and organizations have supported its creation. In particular we thank the contributors for their hard work, creativity, friendship and passion for this book. While editing the book we have lived on opposite sides of the planet, in Australia and Iceland. Meeting to work together on the book has therefore required extensive travel. Our respective universities have provided the support that has enabled us to do this. The University of Iceland awarded Rannveig a research semester and a travel grant in the spring of 2001, which allowed her to spend time in Australia to work with Kelley on conceptualizing and creating the foundations for this book project. In 2004 the Royal Melbourne Institute of Technology University provided financial support for Kelley to travel to Iceland to finish the editing of the book. We owe much thanks for this support; without it the book would not have been possible.

Many people have contributed to our thinking and work on this project. We particularly acknowledge our colleagues Jan Walmsley and Dorothy Atkinson at The Open University for ongoing collaboration and interest in our work. Rannveig also thanks the Open University for awarding her the post of Visiting Research Professor in the spring semester of 2004 and for creating space for her to work on this book. The Social History of Learning Disability Group at the OU provided an inspiring and supportive environment. The stay at the OU was made possible by a research semester awarded to Rannveig by the University of Iceland. When Rannveig first started working with Tom Allen on his life history she was at the Center on Human Policy, Syracuse University, USA. This work was, in part, supported through a subcontract with the Research and Training Center on Community Living, University of Minnesota, supported by the US Department of Education, Office of Special Education and Rehabilitative Services, National Institute on Disability and Rehabilitation Research (NIDRR), through Contract No. H133B031116. Rannveig gratefully acknowledges this support and is particularly thankful to Steven J. Taylor, Director of the Center on Human Policy, and other people at the Center for their friendship and support of her work. Rannveig also thanks the University of Iceland Research Fund and Rannís, the Icelandic Centre for Research, for supporting this project. Kelley would like to thank in particular Millie Mitchell for her thoughtful reflections on some of the chapters in this book. Rannveig thanks Hanna Björg Sigurjónsdóttir and Hrefna K. Oskarsdóttir at the University of Iceland for ongoing support and patience when other work took second place.

Bob Williams, US poet, disabled policy analyst and activist, gave permission to use two of his poems in Chapter 23. Karl Gudmundsson, an Icelandic artist, allowed us to use his artwork for the cover design. We thank both of them. Finally, our gratitude to Vicky Cribb for her valuable assistance with copy editing and to our publisher Jessica Kingsley for her interest and commitment to this project, and her patience and support in working with us.

Kelley Johnson and Rannveig Traustadóttir
Melbourne and Reykjavík, February 2005

Introduction

In and Out of Institutions

Rannveig Traustadóttir, Iceland,
and Kelley Johnson, Australia

This book is about deinstitutionalization. We thought it was important to write about this issue from the point of view of people with intellectual disabilities so that we can understand better what it has meant to them. People with intellectual disabilities, their family members and those who work with them have come together to write about what it has been like to live in large institutions, move out of them and live in the community. The book also looks at new ideas and practices that might make life better for people with intellectual disabilities in the future.

The chapters in this book show that while life in institutions was difficult for many people, institutions were most often set up with good intentions. We think it is important to understand this in order to make sure that community living for people with intellectual disabilities gives people the best possible life. While the people who have written chapters in this book do not want to go back to the institutions, they do talk about some of the problems that they face with living in the community. Sometimes their lives are good; people talk about meeting up with families, working, going on holidays and doing fun things. But they also talk about loneliness and not having meaningful work or choices in their lives.

It seems to be very important that, for community living to work, people with intellectual disabilities have good advocates and other people listen to what they have to say about themselves and what they want. When people have high needs for support or if their behaviour is difficult there is a particular risk that they will find themselves in new kinds of institutions. The book also contains stories about people who have found a home back in their own culture or close to their families and who have a good life in the community.

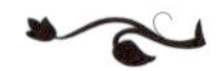

Personal beginnings

Books have particular personal and professional meanings for those who write them. That is also the case with this book. It has emerged from a tangle of professional and personal needs, interests and commitments that have confronted us over many decades of working and advocating with people with intellectual disabilities. We start with these personal beginnings.

Kelley writes: In my office at home there is a small picture of a large institution for people with intellectual disabilities. It was given to me because I was one of a team of people who were involved in the closure of that particular institution. The picture is attractive. In the foreground are green spaces, the sky is blue and the main building of the institution, which was built in 'Dutch colonial style', is painted at an angle. Stairs lead up to the front door and the roofline is elegant and interesting. It looks like a stately home, ready for weekend visitors. Although the etching was made before the institution closed, there are no people walking on the stairs, looking out of the windows or peering over the wall. Where are the 450 people who lived there?

The picture is an idealized image of the institution I knew. For the artist and for some who view it, it holds a particular set of meanings: safety, security, beauty, peace. These are far from my experience of the institution. The picture cannot convey the smells of institutional care; the rituals, the relationships and the pain (and less often the joy) that many people experienced in their lives there. It does not show the steaming pipes that ran overhead across the grounds carrying heating and hissing their way from unit to unit. It does not show the laundry bags piled outside each unit to be picked up and carried away. It does not show the abandoned tram at the back of the grounds where residents found escape from the gaze of staff and some small opportunity for intimacy. The picture shows one face of the institution: solid, built to last for centuries, an attractive entrance for those who arrived, frightened and anxious with their relatives.

The gap between the artist's representation and the actuality of life in a total institution has haunted me over the last ten years. It seems to symbolize the uneasy relationship between the hopes and dreams of good lives for people with intellectual disabilities and the reality: not only in the past but in the present. This book is part of my journey to understand this relationship better and to take some steps to bring the ideal and the reality closer together.

Rannveig writes: During the school holidays when I was 15 years old, I got a summer job in an institution for people with intellectual disabilities. This was in the late 1960s. The routines and living conditions in the institution were a far cry from what ordinary people would recognize as minimally acceptable. Overcrowding, lack of privacy, inhumane treatment and abuse were everyday realities. What I remember most vividly when first entering the institution were the smell and the noises. I was horrified. After a while I got used to the smell and got to know the people who lived in the institution. They were interesting and lovely people and I quickly became fond of them, especially the children. I was bewildered by the inhumanity of the institution. I was only 15 and could not understand how we, as a society, could treat people this way. I made a commitment to do something about it. The only thing I could think of at the time was to try to improve life in the institution. Instead of going back to the education I had planned, I decided to get professional training so I could work with people with disabilities.

This book is part of my initial commitment to improving the lives of people who lived in institutions. However, there is also a more particular reason for writing the book. It is the fulfilment of a promise made to a friend, Tom Allen, who spent more than 60 years in institutions. He struggled all his life to find a place in the community and a family of his own. Sadly, he only managed to find a marginalized place outside the institutions towards the end of his life. When I met Tom he had recently moved out of the institution and did not have many years left to live. In many ways Tom felt as if his life had been wasted in the institutions and the only thing he had to offer was the story of his life. His final wish was for his story to be known in the hope it would help others labelled as having disabilities to lead a better life than he had led. During the last two years of his life I helped document his story and promised I would try to have it published. This book fulfils that promise. Tom was a remarkable man who survived institutional life with dignity and without becoming bitter or broken. His story is a moving and powerful testimony that weaves together the different parts of this book.

A new book on deinstitutionalization?

We began to conceptualize this book with considerable trepidation. After all, there is a large body of literature documenting deinstitutionalization. Personal commitments, promises and concerns are insufficient reasons for another book about an issue, although they are very good motivations! However, our survey of the literature revealed that there was a need for a different kind of book on this topic. The early literature on deinstitutionalization focused on the negative aspects of institutional life for people with intellectual disabilities (Blatt and Kaplan 1966; Grynewald 1971; Kugel and Wolfensberger 1969; Morris 1969; Vail 1966; Wolfensberger 1972).

As the movement towards institutional closure gained momentum, books on deinstitutionalization developed sophisticated analyses of the nature of community living and the processes of deinstitutionalization itself (Booth, Simons and Booth 1990; Bruininks and Lakin 1985; Meyer, Peck and Brown 1991; Scheerenberger 1983; Schwartz 1992; Tøssebro 1992; Tøssebro, Aalto and Brusén 1996). More recent books have attempted to explore the impact of deinstitutionalization across cultures from a policy perspective (Mansell and Ericsson 1996) or have critically analysed community life after the closure of institutions (Sandvin 1996; Tøssebro 1997).

An increasing number of books have described issues relating to the inclusion of people with intellectual disabilities in the community (Edgerton 1991; Gustavsson 1999, 2004; Nisbet and Hagner 2000; Ringsby-Jansson 2002; Sandvin 1993; Schwartz 1992; Swain *et al.* 1993; Taylor, Bogdan and Lutfiyya 1995; Tøssebro 2004; Traustadóttir 1996). There are also autobiographical accounts by people with intellectual disabilities which include descriptions of their lives in institutions and in the community (Atkinson, McCarthy and Walmsley 2000; Atkinson and Williams 1990; Barron 1989; Bogdan and Taylor 1982; Lundgren 1993; Potts and Fido 1991; Traustadóttir and Johnson 2000).

However, nowhere could we find an account that brought together the lived experiences of people with intellectual disabilities and their families with reflections on deinstitutionalization. Nor could we find a book that sought to account for the full processes of deinstitutionalization: institutional life, moving out, living in the community and future possibilities. It seemed to us that if we wanted to understand more fully what has been called one of the major policy shifts in the last 30 years (Chenoweth 2000), then such a book was needed.

We were also conscious that as we move into a new century there is a need to review the current directions of deinstitutionalization. We were unclear about whether we were witnessing a straightforward change in the service system from behind institutional walls to community-based services, or a more fundamental shift in the way people with intellectual disabilities are understood and constructed (Gustavsson 1996). We were also aware that deinstitutionalization has itself changed focus and shape over the past 30 years. In many countries where it has been implemented, it has been subject to wider political and social changes (Sandvin and Söder 1996). The movement in many western countries towards less government intervention, more contractual arrangements in services and a stronger focus on the responsibilities of individuals for their own lives has had a strong impact on deinstitutionalization. In this book we have sought to explore these issues, not from a policy perspective but from the positions of people with intellectual disabilities, their families and service providers.

As the contributors began to send in their chapters we became aware of a number of emerging themes which justified our original intuition that this book would make a unique contribution to our understanding of deinstitutionalization and the lives of people with intellectual disabilities. Some of these themes will be highlighted in a later section of this chapter.

Organization of the book

The overarching theme of the book is how people in different countries and from different perspectives have experienced deinstitutionalization. It also explores implications of deinstitutionalization for them and their communities. In all, 26 authors from seven countries have contributed to this book. Almost half of the chapters are contributions from people with intellectual disabilities (eight chapters) and their family members (three chapters). These chapters are based on a life-story approach and give a unique personal account of the lived experience of institutional life and deinstitutionalization by the people who were subject to it.

The organization of the book reflects the key steps towards deinstitutionalization as it has been experienced by many people with intellectual disabilities: living inside total institutions, moving out, living in the community and moving on to new forms of both institutionalization and community life. The life story of Tom Allen, who was born in 1912 and died in 1991, weaves through the book, providing a powerful testimony of the way institutions and deinstitutionalization have affected one individual over almost a century.

Each of the book's four parts consists of chapters by people with intellectual disabilities or those close to them and by researchers focusing on specific issues and challenges of deinstitutionalization. Some people with intellectual disabilities were unable to write their chapters alone and have done so in collaboration with a researcher. At the beginning of these chapters there is a brief description of how the person's story was written. In other instances ethnographic or qualitative research has been used to document a person's story when he or she was unable to tell it him- or herself. Each part of the book concludes with a reflective chapter written by a person with extensive knowledge and experience of deinstitutionalization who has had access to and considered the preceding chapters. The last chapter of the book, 'Out of the Institution Trap' by John O'Brien, draws together many of the themes of the book, bringing it to a powerful and thoughtful close. By organizing the book this way we wanted, as much as possible, to provide a coherent, reflective account of the processes of deinstitutionalization, based on the experiences of the people most affected by it.

A note on terminology

There is no unity or shared agreement on terminology about disability. Different cultures and countries use different concepts to refer to the people who are the focus of this book. Even in countries where English is the majority language, the terminology is different and politically contested (Eayrs, Ellis and Jones 1993). The most common terms used in English-speaking countries to refer to the people in this book are: learning difficulties, learning disabilities (UK), mental retardation, developmental disabilities (USA) and intellectual disability (Australia and New Zealand). Terminology in other languages is equally varied and complicated, and often difficult to translate over to English.

Debates and differences on disability terminology can be found both inside and outside the disabled people's movements and among disability scholars. The term preferred by most of those who follow a social model of disability is 'disabled people'. Activists and academics who use this term argue that it shifts the focus away from the individual to the experience of oppression by disabling environments. Those arguing this view claim that the term 'people with disabilities' implies that disability is inherent to the individual, rather than locating its cause in social arrangements (Morris 1993; Oliver and Barnes 1998). Others prefer 'people with disabilities', which is also often referred to as 'people-first language'. This term is favoured by most people with intellectual disabilities, their argument being that they want to be called 'people first' and not be named first by their impairment (Clement 2003). In doing this, they also want to assert their common humanity which has sometimes been cast in doubt.

In this book, we have chosen to use the term 'people with intellectual disabilities' for two reasons. First, 'intellectual disability' is the terminology most commonly recognized internationally and is increasingly becoming the term used by international associations and organizations. This is also, in our opinion, the term least likely to create confusion in non-English speaking cultures as to which group of people we are focusing on in this book. Second, we use 'people-first language' as it is consistent with the wishes of many of the contributors.

A note on language and accessibility

We are both strongly committed to making this book as accessible as possible to people with intellectual disabilities. When asking for contributions we asked authors to write in accessible language as much as possible. Despite these efforts, we were conscious that much of the book would remain inaccessible or difficult to negotiate for large numbers of people with intellectual disabilities. In order to make the book accessible to as many people as possible, we also requested that each author write a short plain English summary which appears at the beginning of each chapter. This method proved very successful in an earlier book by and about women with intellectual disabilities (Traustadóttir and Johnson 2000). We are aware that this will not solve all problems of accessibility as there will still be many people who will find the book difficult to access. It is our hope that they will be provided with support to read it. In the meantime, those of us who are writing and researching in the field of intellectual disability need to explore more accessible ways of reporting our work.

Emerging themes

In this section we discuss some of the themes which have emerged from the different parts of the book. We offer these in the introduction as our reflections but are conscious that many other themes can be drawn from the chapters.

Part I: Living Inside

This first part of the book documents the lives of people with intellectual disabilities who were placed in institutions and who spent much of their lives there. The chapters in Part I challenge our views about what intellectual disability is and how it has been historically defined. Tom Allen spent most of his life in institutions for people with intellectual disabilities and was labelled in various ways in his institutional records: as a 'cripple' due to 'infantile paralysis', as having 'mental retardation', being an 'imbecile' and 'having IQ of 37'. Later in his life the institutional records identify him as having 'borderline mental retardation' and finally conclude that he is 'non-mentally retarded'. Tom's own account suggests that he was a thoughtful man who, in difficult circumstances, sought to lead a 'reflective life' and to manage it as best he could.

While Tom's story is perhaps the most directly confronting in the book in terms of the way intellectual disability has been defined, other chapters also reveal the contested nature of this term. Some people continued to live in institutions, not because of their disability but because they were useful; that is, necessary to the maintenance of institutional life. In at least one of the chapters staff opposed a woman leaving the institution because of her skills and hard work as an unpaid worker (see Ingiborg Geirsdóttir's story in Chapter 9 in Part II). At the same time, even when people had more clearly defined disabilities, the reasons for their life in institutions remain problematic. The women who lived in a locked unit (see Kelley Johnson's Chapter 3) were there ostensibly not because of their 'intellectual disability' but because management decided that they were a risk to themselves or to others; in short, they were uncontainable women. Their 'challenging behaviour' was not seen as something that may have been due, at least in part, to their life experiences but was seen as integral to intellectual disability.

The chapters in Part I reveal that it was poverty, abuse and family problems that led many people to leave the community and be placed in institutions. In our view not enough weight has been given to these issues in considering both people's institutional lives and their subsequent lives in the community.

This part of the book also raises the question: who were the institutions for? Jan Walmsley (Chapter 2) gives a historical account of institutions which seeks to demystify and mediate the demonization these places have been subject to during deinstitutionalization. She does not offer an apologia for institutions – far from it – but her chapter clarifies some of the motivations of those who were involved in establishing institutions and the often complex relationships that existed between them, residents and families. There was an ongoing tension within institutions between the need to care for and protect people with intellectual disabilities and the efforts to control and exclude them as possible dangers to the wider community.

As we have moved to an era of community living for people with intellectual disabilities, it is salutary to reflect on how little this tension has changed. Those who remained longest in the institutions were those with higher needs for support, were older and were judged 'most risky'. With the increasing emphasis on rights for people with intellectual disabilities, the focus on care has shifted to one of inclusion. It would seem that this, like the preceding care ethic, remains problematic and difficult to attain (Philpot and Ward 1995; Ramcharan, Grant and Borland 1997; Ward 1998). However, it can also be argued that we have translated the control previously exerted on people through locked doors and high walls into the more subtle discourse of risk management with its rituals of assessment and strategic placement (Rose 1998, 2000; Johnson and Tait 2003).

While there are accounts throughout this book of warm relationships between residents in institutions and staff members, they form a background to the often scalding memories of repeated abuse and neglect of people with intellectual disabilities by carers. The writers do not locate such abuse with one individual or seek retribution or justice. Rather, the abuse seems to be recognized by the contributors to this book as something that was part of the system. It had to be borne rather than resisted. The consequences of systemic abuse and neglect described in so many chapters in this book reach their climax in Ian Freckelton's account (in Chapter 4) of the unnecessary and tragic deaths of nine men living in a large institution.

Other chapters suggest that it is simplistic to locate such abuse within the institutional system and to believe that it is solely a function of 'managing' large groups of people in often difficult circumstances. Given the widespread nature of such abuse it is more useful to locate systemic abuse and its consequences within the discourses of intellectual disability itself. Over a period of almost a hundred years, a body of generally accepted knowledge has been developed about people with intellectual disabilities and then put into practice to shape their treatment and their lives.

Many people with intellectual disabilities are dependent on others for varying levels of support, whether it is within institutional walls or in the community, and they often find it difficult to articulate their experiences. People who are isolated from others are particularly vulnerable to projected fears and frustrations experienced by those who support them. In the light of the chapters in this book we do need to ask seriously whether the rhetoric of deinstitutionalization is sufficient to alter the discourses which have placed people with intellectual disabilities in this position. We need to ask what training staff (who often worked in institutions) have received that will lead them to challenge and question their anxieties and fears.

Resistance is one of the themes that runs through the book and reflects the fact that people with intellectual disabilities used different ways to protest about their situation. They spoke up, became angry, hid, ran away, took their cases to court, fought, exhibited 'challenging' or 'bad' behaviours and found support from others, to name but a few manifestations of resistance. But there are also examples of how people 'gave in' or changed strategies over to a more 'co-operative' mode in order to survive because of the severity of the possible consequences of resistance. It is easy to attribute powerlessness and victimhood to people with intellectual disabilities in the face of the abuse many received. However, it is apparent from chapters in this book that some people made conscious decisions not to protest about their treatment because of anxieties about the effects of such complaints on themselves and those around them. Fear of the consequences was certainly well founded and played a part in the decision-making.

Some writers in this book did not resist or protest about their treatment because they were protecting those around them. People who have written chapters for this book show concern for their families; for example Tom Allen did not tell his family what his life was really like in the institution because he did want not to add to his family's guilt about sending him to the institution and excluding him from their lives. Seeing people with intellectual disabilities as active and often silent decision-makers in their own lives can fundamentally shift the way they are viewed. They are neither heroes nor victims but, rather, they make decisions in the context of their families and social lives, as we all do.

Part II: Moving Out

This part of the book is concerned with the often overlooked experience of actually moving out of the institution. In Chapter 8, Chris Bigby reveals the complexity of planning and design that underlies each institutional closure. Yet when some people with intellectual disabilities write about the experience of deinstitutionalization, moving out is not mentioned. They write and speak vividly of the institution and of their life in the community, as if one day they lived in the institution and the next they lived outside. Perhaps this is because they have not been included in the planning processes.

As Jan Tøssebro notes (Part III, Chapter 16), people with intellectual disabilities often do not have a voice about the important decisions: where and with whom they will live and the kinds of supports they will receive. There may also be other explanations. As observers of institutional closure we found that the actual process created anxiety and was stressful for all those who took part in it, but particularly for the people who lived at the institution (Johnson 1998). People with whom they had lived left suddenly and unexpectedly, and services they had used were closed down. They walked past silent units and wards which once had been their homes and they lived with strangers. Perhaps moving out is like the experience of birth. People forget its pain in the new outcomes of parenthood or infancy. Similarly, the stress of moving may be lost in the new lives people have in the community.

There is not, however, a total silence about moving out. For some people it was a struggle they had to win against families, staff or advocates. In Chapter 7 Tom Allen writes graphically of the court case that preceded his move to the community and in Chapter 9 Ingiborg Geirsdóttir tells of the sterilization that was a necessary prerequisite to her leaving the institution.

Most troubling in this part of the book is how people with intellectual disabilities remain subject to management rather than being individuals with preferences and particular needs during the process of institutional closure. A 'place' in the community is offered but it is not necessarily the kind of home the person needs or wants. There are few or no choices offered to people about their future lives and the focus seems to continue to be on structured programmes and kinds of services rather than on any detailed exploration with the person about his or her dreams, wishes and desires. Limited resources and having to manage large groups of people in transition may partially explain this. However, the process has some uncomfortable echoes of institutional experiences many people had lived with in the past. It continues the dependency on others and the sense of not being an active agent in one's own life.

All of us find it difficult at times to articulate our desires. It must be especially difficult for some people with intellectual disabilities to express preferences for a lifestyle they have not experienced. But some of the writers in this book make clear their preferences even when they cannot speak. For example, in Chapter 10, Rowan, who cannot tell his needs, finds ways to show his family what he wants. One of the problems encountered by some writers in the book is the lack of the ability or willingness of those around them actually to hear what they are saying.

In this book at least, those who have listened to the voices and preferences of people with intellectual disabilities have tended to be family members and, in far fewer instances, a staff member supporting the person. Yet families' agendas can be mixed and at times run counter to the interests and needs of the person with a disability. We need, it seems, some careful processes in place to ensure that those around people with intellectual disabilities are sensitized to hearing them.

Life does not always give us what we want but usually we are able to find reasons for why this is so. Too many times in this book desires and needs are denied without reason. Why should Ingiborg be sterilized, for instance? Why did Tom have to live with someone he did not like? Why was it so difficult for people to retain old relationships after moving from an institution?

Part III: Living Outside

None of the chapters in Part III reflects a person's desire to return to institutional life and, in most aspects, people's lives improved in the community. There are accounts of fishing trips (Emil in Chapter 14), of renewed contacts with families (Vicki in Chapter 15) and of peaceful lives, work and play (Victor in Chapter 13). The lives people write about are quiet, and seemingly minor incidents are recalled and recounted with great vividness. It is likely that when people have largely been denied participation in the significant issues of life – love, work, births and deaths – each deviation from the usual gains enormous importance. However, this does not mean that everyone found happiness in the community and there are accounts which reveal that life in the community can be difficult. In Chapter 15, Jen Devers writes of her sister's continuing problems to find a place there, even while she records the happiness of renewed family contacts. And for some, the threat of reinstitutionalization remains a shadow, a fear or a nightmare, as Tom Allen describes so vividly in Chapter 12.

The importance of family to people with intellectual disabilities is a recurrent theme in this book and is particularly relevant in Part III. Families support, advocate and provide spaces away from the sense of still being different, devalued and the recipient of services. Families come together for the special events of the year and share the celebrations of birthdays, Christmas and other important events. The vividness with which these events are recalled by people suggests the profound sense of deprivation and abandonment they have previously felt due to their being excluded or isolated from their families.

An important issue raised in a number of the chapters is the erosion of initial enthusiasm and energy that is there soon after leaving the institution. The bright hopes that were held for an alternative lifestyle for Rowan (Chapter 10) gradually disappeared. Jen Devers (Chapter 15) found that the initial excitement that was attached to her sister's reappearance in the community soon changed to a series of struggles and conflicts with staff and other service providers. Tom Allen (Chapter 12) expresses disappointment at the lack of freedom, activities and comfort in his new life. The hopes and dreams of a better world outside the institution that sustained some people with intellectual disabilities throughout their institutional lives are confronted by a continuing isolation and exclusion from 'real' community life. There are lessons here in looking back to institutions. Many were founded with high aspirations and ideals. They were to provide opportunities for people with intellectual disabilities. It took almost 100 years for them to be recognized as offering at best custodial care and at worst an abusive environment. It is important now to think of ways to prevent a similar degeneration in the brave new world of the community.

Proponents of deinstitutionalization have positioned institutions as 'all bad' and the community as 'all good'. The accounts in this book suggest that while the community is better than the institution, it does not match up either to hopes or to the realities of the lives that most of us live, as Jan Tøssebro articulates eloquently in Chapter 16.

Part IV: Moving On

In the last part of the book, Part IV, we consider the themes that are currently emerging in deinstitutionalization and community life. There are hopeful glimpses of a future where people with intellectual disabilities are seen as individuals within their own culture and are included within it (see, for example, Chapters 20 and 22). In many services there is an increased focus on rights and on participation. However, many of the old themes of control and surveillance that permeated institutional life have been reconstructed in the community. This is particularly so for those who continue to be seen as a 'risk'. There seems to be a serious lack of new ideas about how to create alternative options for people who fall into this category. Rather, new kinds of institutions or heightened surveillance continue to provide the 'solutions', as Gardner and Glanville describe in Chapter 19.

Further, just as it took scandals and testimonies of abuse to close many large institutions, now crises and problems experienced by people with intellectual disabilities are the motivations for change in community services. For example, Tom only received his long-desired companionship and freedom when he was dying. The chapters also reveal that unless someone is advocating for an individual, life goes on in similar ways whether one is in institutions or out of them. It seems to us significant that the people in this book who have found satisfying lives in the community have had strong advocates who have known them well, taken up their issues and have had the resources to try out new ideas. The lives of the first generation of people with intellectual disabilities in Sweden who have grown up without the existence of institutions, described by Magnus Tideman in Chapter 18, reveal that problems of social isolation and lack of meaning in people's lives continue to be major themes. Bricks and mortar are relatively easy to tear down and build. It is much more difficult to find ways of supporting people so that they can have meaningful lives that are akin to those of other citizens.

In Chapter 21 Paul Cambridge explains some of the dilemmas that this part of the book exposes. He places deinstitutionalization in a wider social context. Changes in the way governments do their business, the movement to contractualism and the subsequent fragmentation of services in many countries sometimes make it more difficult to develop innovative ways that will assist people with intellectual disabilities to lead satisfying and meaningful lives.

Conclusion

We entitled this book *Deinstitutionalization and People with Intellectual Disabilities: In and Out of Institutions.* The title became more apt as we read the contributions to the book. Deinstitutionalization is not something that happens once in a person's life. In almost all the chapters in this book people with intellectual disabilities have moved in and out of some form of institutional care throughout their lives. This movement occurs in reality but it also exists as a fear and a continuing nightmare for many people who are now living in the community.

We hope this book will provide an opportunity for readers to reflect not only on the transitions involved in deinstitutionalization but also upon how we understand the subjectivity of the people with intellectual disabilities who have experienced it. Without this kind of reflection we run the risk of recreating an institutional way of life for people as they move into the community.

References

Atkinson, D., McCarthy, M., Walmsley, J., Cooper, M., Rolph, S. and Barette, P. (2000) *Good Times Bad Times: Women with Learning Difficulties Telling their Stories.* Kidderminster: BILD.

Atkinson, D. and Williams, F. (eds) (1990) *'Know Me as I am': An Anthology of Prose, Poetry and Art by People with Learning Difficulties.* London: Hodder and Stoughton.

Barron, D. (1989) 'Locked away: Life in an institution.' In A. Brechin and J. Walmsley (eds) *Making Connections: Reflections on the Lives and Experiences of People with Learning Difficulties.* London: Hodder and Stoughton.

Blatt, B. and Kaplan, F. (1966) *Christmas in Purgatory: A Photographic Essay on Mental Retardation.* Boston: Allyn & Bacon.

Bogdan, R. and Taylor, S.J. (1982) *Inside Out: The Meaning of Mental Retardation.* Toronto: University of Toronto Press.

Booth, T., Simons, K. and Booth, W. (1990) *Outward Bound: Relocation and Community Care for People with Learning Difficulties.* Milton Keynes: Open University Press.

Bruininks, R.H. and Lakin, K.C. (eds) (1985) *Living and Learning in the Least Restrictive Environment.* Baltimore, MD: Paul H. Brookes.

Chenoweth, L. (2000) 'Closing the doors: Insights and reflections on deinstitutionalisation.' In M. Jones and L.A.B. Marks (eds) *Explorations on Law and Disability in Australia.* Melbourne: The Federation Press.

Clement, T. (2003) 'An Ethnography of People First Anytown: A Description, Analysis, and Interpretation of an Organizational Culture.' Unpublished PhD dissertation. Milton Keynes: Open University.

Eayrs, C.B., Ellis, N. and Jones, R.S.P. (1993) 'Which label? An investigation into the effects of terminology on public perceptions of and attitudes towards people with learning difficulties.' *Disability Handicap and Society 8*, 2, 111–117.

Edgerton, R. (1991) *Lives of Older People with Mental Retardation in the Community.* Baltimore, MD: Paul H. Brookes.

Grynewald, K. (ed.) (1971) *Menneskemanipulering på totalinstitutisjoner: Fra dehumanisering til normalisering* ('Human manipulation in total institutions: From dehumanization to normalization'). Taning & Appels Forlag.

Gustavsson, A. (1996) 'Reforms and everyday meanings of intellectual disability.' In J. Tøssebro, A. Gustavsson and G. Dyrendahl (eds) *Intellectual Disabilities in the Nordic Welfare States: Policies and Everyday Life.* Oslo: Norwegian Academic Press.

Gustavsson, A. (1999) *Inifrån utanförskapet* ('From within the outsidership'). Lund: Studentlitteratur.

Gustavsson, A. (2004) *Delaktighetens språk* ('The language of participation'). Lund: Studentlitteratur.

Johnson, K. (1998) *Deinstitutionalising Women: An Ethnographic Study of Institutional Closure.* Melbourne: Cambridge University Press.

Johnson, K. and Tait, S. (2003) 'Throwing away the key: People with intellectual disabilities and involuntary detention.' In I. Freckelton and K. Diesfeld (eds) *Involuntary Detention and Civil Commitment: International Perspectives.* London: Bloomsbury.

Kugel, R.B. and Wolfensberger, W. (eds) (1969) *Changing Patterns in Residential Services for the Mentally Retarded.* Washington, DC: President's Committee on Mental Retardation.

Lundgren, K. (1993) *Åke's Book.* Stockholm: Riksforbudet FUB (The Swedish National Association for Persons with Mental Handicap).

Mansell, J. and Ericsson, K. (1996) *Deinstitutionalisation and Community Living: Intellectual Disability Services in Britain, Scandinavia, and the USA.* London: Chapman & Hall.

Meyer, L.H., Peck, C.A. and Brown, L. (eds) (1991) *Critical Issues in the Lives of People with Severe Disabilities.* Baltimore, MD: Paul H. Brookes.

Morris, J. (1993) *Independent Lives? Community Care and Disabled People.* Basingstoke: Macmillan.

Morris, P. (1969) *Put Away: A Sociological Study of Institutions for the Mentally Retarded.* London: Routledge and Kegan Paul.

Nisbet, J. and Hagner, D. (eds) (2000) *Part of the Community: Strategies for Including Everyone.* Baltimore, MD: Paul H. Brookes.

Oliver, M. and Barnes, C. (1998) *Disabled People and Social Policy: From Exclusion to Inclusion.* London: Longman.

Philpot, T. and Ward, L. (eds) (1995) *Values and Visions: Changing Ideas in Services for People with Learning Difficulties.* Oxford: Butterworth Heinemann.

Potts, M. and Fido, R. (1991) *A Fit Person to be Removed: Personal Accounts of Life in a Mental Deficiency Institution.* Plymouth: Northcote House.

Ramcharan, P., Grant, G. and Borland, J. (eds) (1997) *Empowerment in Everyday Life: Learning Disability.* London: Jessica Kingsley Publishers.

Ringsby-Jansson, B. (2002) *Vardagslivets arenor: Om människor med utvecklingsstörning, deras vardag och sociala liv* ('Arenas of everyday life: About people with intellectual disabilities and their everyday and social life'). Göteborg: Institutionen för socialt arbete, Göteborgs universitet.

Rose, N. (1998) 'Governing risky individuals: The role of psychiatry in new regimes of control.' *Psychiatry, Psychology and Law 3*, 2, 177–95.

Rose, N. (2000) *Powers of Freedom: Reframing Political Thought.* Cambridge: Cambridge University Press.

Sandvin, J.T. (ed.) (1993) *Mot normalt: Omsorgsideologier i forandring* ('Towards a normal life: Changing care ideologies'). Oslo: Kommunalforlaget.

Sandvin, J.T. (1996) 'The transition to community services in Norway.' In J. Mansell and K. Ericsson (eds) *Deinstitutionalisation and Community Living: Intellectual Disability Services in Britain, Scandinavia and the USA.* London: Chapman & Hall.

Sandvin, J. and Söder, M. (1996) 'Welfare state reconstruction.' In J. Tøssebro, A. Gustavsson and G. Dyrendahl (eds) *Intellectual Disabilities in the Nordic Welfare States: Policies and Everyday Life.* Oslo: Norwegian Academic Press.

Schwartz, D.B. (1992) *Crossing the River: Creating a Conceptual Revolution in Community and Disability.* Cambridge, MA: Brookline Books.

Sheerenberger, R.C. (1983) *A History of Mental Retardation.* Baltimore, MD: Paul H. Brookes.

Swain, J., Finkelstein, V., French, S. and Oliver, M. (eds) (1993) *Disabling Barriers – Enabling Environments.* London: Sage.

Taylor, S.J., Bogdan, R. and Lutfiyya, Z.M. (eds) (1995) *The Variety of Community Experience: Qualitative Studies of Family and Community Life.* Baltimore, MD: Paul H. Brookes.

Tøssebro, J. (1992) *Institusjonsliv i velferdsstaten: Levekår under HVPU-reformen* ('Institutions in the welfare state: Living conditions of people with intellectual disabilities'). Oslo: ad Notam Gyldendal.

Tøssebro, J. (ed.) (1997) *Den vanskelige integreringen* ('The difficult integration'). Oslo: Universitetsforlaget.

Tøssebro, J. (ed.) (2004) *Integrering och inkludering* ('Integration and inclusion'). Lund: Studentlitteratur.

Tøssebro, J., Aalto, M. and Brusén, P. (1996) 'Changing ideologies and patterns of services: The Nordic countries.' In J. Tøssebro, A. Gustavsson and G. Dyrendahl (eds) *Intellectual Disabilities in the Nordic Welfare States: Policies and Everyday Life.* Oslo: Norwegian Academic Press.

Tøssebro, J. and Kittelsaa, A. (eds) (2004) *Exploring the Living Conditions of Disabled People.* Lund: Studentlitteratur.

Traustadóttir, R. (1996) 'Everyday life in the community.' In J. Tøssebro, A. Gustavsson and G. Dyrendahl (eds) *Intellectual Disabilities in the Nordic Welfare States: Policies and Everyday Life.* Oslo: Norwegian Academic Press.

Traustadóttir, R. and Johnson, K. (eds) (2000) *Women with Intellectual Disabilities: Finding a Place in the World.* London: Jessica Kingsley Publishers.

Vail, D. (1966) *Dehumanization and the Institutional Career.* Springfield, IL: C.C. Thomas.

Ward, L. (ed.) (1998) *Innovations in Advocacy and Empowerment for People with Intellectual Disabilities.* Chorley: Lisieux Hall Publications.

Wolfensberger, W. (1972) *The Origin and Nature of our Institutional Models.* Syracuse, NY: Human Policy Press.

PART I

Living Inside

1

Sixty Years in the Institution

Thomas F. Allen with Rannveig Traustadóttir
and Lisa Spina, USA

My name is Tom Allen. I was born in 1912. I was first sent to an institution when I was two or three years old. When I was six years old I became very sick and was sent home because the people in the institution thought I was going to die and they wanted me to die at home. My mother nursed me back to health and I stayed at home with my family. I was the next youngest of seven children. We were poor but we always had plenty of food. We were a large happy family. Then my mother died suddenly. My father married again and they could not take care of me at home and sent me to the institution again when I was 15 years old. I was only meant to be there for a year or two but I ended up spending 45 years in this institution called Rome State School.

I did not like being in the institution. I felt like no one cared about me. I felt all alone in the world, angry and hurt. I was desperate. No one in the institution understood me and the staff punished me for my behaviours. I was sent to the back ward with the most disabled people. This was supposed to be a punishment but it turned out well. I liked some of the staff and they liked me. I worked a lot on this ward. It was good because it gave me something to do with my time. There was little else to do on the ward. Most of the time I spent at Rome the patients (as we were called at the time) were not allowed to go off the wards, except for special occasions like when family came for a visit.

I had been in Rome for five years when my family came for a visit for the first time. It was *so* good to see them. I had gotten a few letters from some of my brothers and sisters so I had a pretty good idea of how everyone was doing.

After having been in Rome State School for 45 years I went to another institution: Craig Developmental Center. There was nothing to do there and I was terribly bored. About a month before I left Craig I got my own room. It was the first and only time I have had a room all to myself. I liked having the privacy.

In 1982 I moved to Syracuse Developmental Center at the age of 69. There were some good things about Syracuse, it was a new building so it did not smell too bad. I also got involved with self-advocacy. But I was tired of the institutions and wanted to move out. I wanted a home before I died. I did not want to die in the institution.

Rannveig and Lisa write: Tom began writing his story long before he met the two of us. He started it in the 1970s while still living in the institution. In the beginning he wrote it to have something to do during long empty days. As time went by his views changed and he felt more and more compelled to tell the story of his life. The feeling that his life had been wasted grew stronger and he saw his story as a way of accomplishing something and leaving something behind. Tom also realized that he was one of the few people his age who had managed to tell his story. It could therefore be a testimony for so many others who were never heard.

It was an enormous effort for Tom to tell his story. He had limited use of his arms and could not write the story himself, so he had to dictate it to other people who wrote it down. Tom had difficulties speaking. He spoke very slowly, could only say a couple of words at a time and his words were often hard to understand.

Dictating his story to other people was therefore a very, very slow process. Because Tom could not speak in whole sentences, the people assisting him had to compose the sentences and read them back to him to make sure the wording was the way Tom wanted. The first part of the story was written while he lived in the institutions with the assistance of staff members who were his friends. After he moved out he continued to work on the story with our assistance. Tom worked very hard on the story the year before he died. As he grew weaker he realized he would not be able to complete it and asked the two of us to finish it for him. To make sure we had full authority to do so, he had his lawyer prepare a statement declaring that he authorized Rannveig Traustadóttir and Lisa Spina to finish his story. Tom did not live to approve the last version of his story. But before he died we had long discussions about how the story should be and he gave us instructions about what should be there, how it should be told and what should be the 'tone' of the story. We have tried our very best to honour his wishes and sincerely hope that he would approve the story we present in this book.

Although Tom spent over 60 years of his life in institutions for people with intellectual disabilities, he did not think of himself in those terms. He saw himself as physically impaired or 'crippled' as he calls it in the story. The institutional records describe him in different ways at different times. When he was readmitted to Rome State School in 1928 he was said to have an IQ of 37, when he moved into Craig Developmental Center in 1973 his records describe him as having 'borderline mental retardation' and in 1979 his records say he is 'non-mentally retarded'.

For more information about the background to Tom's story and how it was written, we refer people to the Epilogue to Tom Allen's life story on p.274.

Tom's story

My name is Thomas Fredrick Allen. Everybody calls me Tom for short. I was born on 1 November, 1912 in Canisteo, a small town in New York. I was born normal but when I was two years old I got polio which left me crippled[1] and hard to understand. My family was poor and I was the sixth child. As I recall, when I got sick my mother had a nervous breakdown and the doctors sent her to Willard, a mental hospital, for two months. In the meantime I was sent to Rome State School.[2] I was two or three years old at the time. I was at Rome for four or five years. I don't remember the stay there clearly because I was so little but I remember being put on different wards for rehabilitation. I could only crawl on my hands and knees. They tried to see what kind of a person I was. I couldn't tell them myself. What I do remember is how hard it was to be sent away from my family. I was alone and scared.

I was about six years old when I went into the hospital building at Rome State School. I had a double pneumonia. The doctor thought I was going to die and sent for my mother. The doctor asked her to take me home because he thought it would be better for me to die at home. My mother went back home and convinced my father to come and get me. She assured him that she could take care of me at home. About two weeks later my dad came and took me home. I was sick and weak but somehow I understood I was going home to my mother. I thought we would never get there. It was a long ride because cars only went 35 miles per hour in those days. We did not get home 'til 1pm the next day.

My father, mother, sisters, brothers, grandmother and a couple of cousins all lived in one big house and everybody was waiting for me. When we got home, my mother grabbed me out of the car, brought me into the house and cleaned me up. I was very tired from the long drive but happy to be home. That night there was quite a celebration. Everybody came to see me – all our friends and neighbours. It was quite a home-coming.

For the next few weeks my mother worried about my pneumonia. She watched over me all the time. The family doctor came to examine me and said I would be all right. I recovered but as a result of this illness my lungs and respiratory system have always been weak. I often get pneumonia and have had asthma for much of my life.

The next years were the happiest of my life. I lived at home with my large and lively family. My mother took care of me. She helped me get dressed each morning, helped me eat, helped me go to the bathroom and do other things I could not do by myself. My mother also took care of my grandmother. She was my mother's mother. Me and my grandma had good times together and sometimes she helped me eat. She was more than 80 years old.

We lived in Canisteo by the freight yard and I used to sit near the window looking out at the railroad tracks. My grandmother sat in her wheelchair beside me. We would sit there by the hour and every time a freight train came by we counted all the different cars. We would pick out the carloads of chickens and things. It was fun trying to remember how many cars there were.

My family

My parents had ten children but only seven lived. My brother Bob was the oldest. He was born in 1903. He was a railroad man. Whenever he wasn't working he used to hunt or fish. I never got along too well with Bob. Every little noise I made would bother him. Thelma was the next oldest. She was two years younger than Bob. I always liked Thelma. She sometimes helped me eat, and she and I used to talk about different things. I felt like I could tell her anything and she understood me. Thelma worked in a factory where they made rulers and yardsticks. In those days the hours were from six o'clock in the morning to five in the afternoon and when she came home she used to help with the housework. All the kids helped.

Marion came after Thelma. She was born in 1907 and was two years younger than Thelma. They used to go out together until Marion got married when she was about 17 years old. Marion lived with her husband in an apartment house over the grocery store in town. She often came over during the week to see everybody. Marion and I always got along very well. She also helped me eat sometimes or helped me with other things.

Dick was next. He was born in 1909. He was a good kid but he was always getting in all kinds of mischief. We got along pretty good. After Dick came Margaret. She died when she was only four months old. I don't know what she died of. I came next. There were a pair of twins after me, but they died at birth.

Neal was the last of the Allens. He was born in 1918. He was an active youngster. We used to play together a lot because he was the only one who was not going to school. Except for occasional fights we always got along. As a child I was closest to Neal and in my adult years Neal was the one who kept the closest contact with me and visited me most often in the institution.

As children, Neal and I used to invent games to play. We used to make believe we were always going somewhere. We'd line up chairs and use them for a train. Of course, my grandmother helped with the game. I used to get on the front of my grandmother's wheelchair. One day we were playing the game and going someplace. I wanted to go too. My brother Neal said, 'I can't take all the cripples and fools'. My mother heard him. She grabbed Neal and gave him a good swat. He was only four or five years old and didn't know better. I was hurt and cried because I did not want to be called names like that.

I guess I was lucky my grandmother used a wheelchair so I was not the only one in the family who could not walk. I don't know why she could not walk but before she became crippled she used to teach school. I was also lucky that she used to be a teacher because she taught me a lot of things. She taught me how to count to 20 and taught me to tell the time of day on our clock. My grandmother also played dominoes with me and she read me all the nursery rhymes. We had fun together and we kept each other company during the long days, especially after Neal started going to school because then it was just the two of us home with mother.

I wished I could go to school like my brothers and sisters but I understood why I couldn't. Mother and grandmother explained to me that crippled children could not go to school. Sometimes my brothers and sisters told me what they learned in school. I often thought about how much I wanted to go there with them and I daydreamed being in school. School was just a dream for me. I never went to school in my whole life. Never. The only education I had was what my grandmother taught me.

At that time I had no wheelchair and had to crawl everywhere I went, or I had to be carried. I didn't go out much and stayed home most of the time.

I have not said much about my mother and father. My mother was always a happy-go-lucky woman. She had a great sense of humour and liked to have fun. She was very sensitive but would not let anyone run over her. She took care of the family. She cooked and cleaned, and the kids helped. She also sewed a lot. We never bought clothes because she made all our clothes. I loved my mother very much. She was the most important person in my life.

My father worked all day in a factory. This was a factory where they made metal sheet signs. If anything went wrong with the machinery he knew what to do to fix it. He was always full of fun – like my mother. Me and my father got along great. He always stuck up for me.

We were poor but we always had plenty of food. My mother used to go shopping every Saturday to get groceries. My father used to go with her. We all lived in a big house with plenty of room. Almost every Sunday we had a houseful of company. Everybody came to see us. We had lots of food and sat around and talked about different things. That was before we had radio or television. All we had was a phonograph – the kind you cranked. When it wound down you had to crank it up again.

On special occasions we'd have a square dance in the house. We invited all our friends and family. These get-togethers would last until two or three in the morning and we had lots of fun. Those were the happy days; the happiest days of my life. Everyone worked hard but we were one happy family right up until 1924.

Family problems

My grandmother died in January 1924. I was 11 years old at the time. She was 84 years old and had leg ulcers. Somehow they got infected and she died. I lost my best friend.

And then came the big blow. My mother died in March that same year. She had been away all day visiting relatives and came home that night kind of tired.

She went to bed about ten o'clock and died in her sleep that night. She had a heart attack. She was only 44 years old. My father woke up and realized what had happened. I was sleeping in the same room. My father grabbed me out of the room and took me to Thelma's room. I didn't know what was going on for a while but Thelma finally told me after about an hour. It was the most difficult moment of my life to hear her say that mother had died.

My father called the doctor but she was already gone. Someone called Marion. Bob was out on the railroad. We got a telegram out to him. It happened so suddenly. I cried like a baby. Neal cried. We all cried together. All our friends and neighbours came. They pitched in and brought things for us to eat. Three days later she was buried in the family plot. Thelma took over after my mother died. She was only 19 years old. Thelma changed the house all around. She put the bedroom where the living room used to be and the living room where the bedroom used to be. It was all different.

In September of 1924 my father got married again. Belle was my stepmother's name. She was married before, and had a boy and a girl of her own. The boy was about my age but he didn't live with us. Arlene was her daughter. She was younger than Neal. Belle's mother lived with us too. Belle took over and her kids came first. Everyone would argue and we just couldn't get along. Bob moved out. Dick joined the army. He left to get away from everybody, especially Belle. They didn't get along at all. Thelma got married.

It seemed everyone had gone. Neal was in school all day and Arlene went to school in the afternoon. It was just Belle, her mother and myself at home, with Dad working all day. Belle was jealous of me; especially of the attention my dad would give me. She was jealous of all us kids. Then my father lost his job and Belle's mother died.

We lived in a small basement apartment and things became worse. Belle got more jealous. My dad tried to make it better but couldn't. Belle said I was too heavy for her to lift and she could not stay home all day to look after me. Belle talked my father into sending me back to Rome State School in 1928. They also thought maybe I'd get some schooling there. Belle and my dad talked to me about it. I sort of agreed with them. I didn't want to be in the way.

I also wanted to go to school and get some education and I was hoping to get an education at Rome. My dad and Belle promised me I'd only be there a year or two.

Back in the institution

I went back to Rome on 15 September 1928. I was 15 years old. We left home about 6am and my father drove our own beat-up car. All I brought with me were the clothes on my back. That was it. You were not allowed to bring any personal belongings. We had two flat tyres on the way. It was just Belle, my father and myself, so father had to fix the flats. We stopped on the way to have lunch.

We arrived at Rome around 1.30 in the afternoon and went to the administration building to admit me. My father had to bring all my papers there. The people in the office said I had to start out by staying in the new admissions ward. A couple of attendants came to the office and carried me over to the ward. I said goodbye to my dad in the administration building. He was not allowed to come to the ward. I felt sad but I didn't cry because I didn't think I was going to be there long.

When we came over to the ward the attendants undressed me and put my clothes away. They gave me a bath and dressed me in hospital clothes: a white pair of pants and a white shirt. After they changed my clothes they had me lie down on a bed and did all kinds of different tests on me. I was in the new admissions ward for about three weeks. Then I was sent to the B-Building. That was a bad move for me. My God, I had more trouble in B-Building than any other building in Rome.

Resisting the institution

I was determined to have my way and wanted to make some of the decisions about what I did and when. The staff did not agree. They made all the decisions and I was supposed to do what they said. I didn't want to obey. I didn't like the staff and I got into a lot of conflict with them. To make things worse the other patients[3] would tell on one another. That's why I was in trouble most of the time. There was a husband-and-wife team looking over the whole ward. All the wards in B-Building had a husband-and-wife team. In those days they worked long hours, between 11 and 14 hours a day. B-Building had only men living in it, men of all age groups. B-Building was for people who were smarter and my ward was for cripples. Most of us needed to use wheelchairs. It was on this ward that I used a wheelchair for the first time. I did not get a chair of my own. I just used one of the wheelchairs on the ward. Later I got my own chair. I learned to push myself around a little with my feet because my arms were not strong enough to push a chair. If I was not in a wheelchair I had a hard time moving around on my own. Still, staff would usually not put me in a wheelchair during the day. Instead, they would put me in a regular chair where I was stuck all day.

There were about 55 patients on the ward. The beds were upstairs in the dormitory, which was one big room. The dormitory held patients from two wards so there were about 100 men sleeping in the same room. We were put to bed about seven o'clock in the evening. The beds were so close that there was just about enough room to walk between them. It was hard to sleep there. It smelled real bad.

We would get up at 5.30 in the morning and spend the day in the day room. Usually they would put me on one side of the day room and leave me there all day. I could look around but that was about all I could do all day. There were no programmes in those days. No school. No work. No physical therapy. No speech therapy. No nothing. I had hoped to get some education in Rome but there was no such thing.

There was a lot of fighting on the ward and I didn't like the violence. It scared me. It has always been difficult for me to deal with conflict. I want people to be friends and be at peace with one another. Rome was not a place for me and I didn't want to be there.

My first years in Rome were the most difficult in my life. I felt like no one understood me nor cared about me. I felt all alone in the world. I was a desperate, angry young man. No one understood my anger and desperation. Instead, I was punished for not behaving – often severely. The staff would, for example, put me on the floor in the back of the bathroom door and I had to lay there all day; sometimes without getting anything to eat.

I was in trouble in B-Building because I was protesting against being in Rome. The time went by. I wanted to go home. I did not have any visitors for the first five years in Rome. I felt abandoned by my family and was very lonely. Like the rest of my family, I have always been very religious. I turned to God. I had nowhere else to turn. I asked God to get me out of there and I prayed that my family would come to visit me. Nothing happened. I became very desperate. I feared that the Lord had left me like my family had. My desperation was so deep it is hard to describe.

On the back ward

After four years I got into serious trouble and I was transferred over to H-Building. I was about 20 or 21 years old at the time. The staff in B-Building thought they were punishing me by moving me, but they did me a great favour instead. The people who lived in H-Building were more disabled and the building was old. It was what you would call a 'back ward'. Living conditions were not as good as in B-Building and we sometimes had bed bugs. Despite this I liked the new ward.

Things began to change for me because I decided I should begin to pick up things for myself. I figured out that if I helped to do things such as sort the laundry, count sheets and pillow cases and stuff like that, I got along better with the staff. They liked me. Once in a while we had squabbles but for the most part we got along. We got along because I thought I'd better change. I got acquainted with one of the staff and I got along pretty well with him. When I had the chance to move to another ward I decided to stay where I got along with people. When they built a new H-Building they also offered me to move but I stayed where I was, but it became known as I-Building. I stayed on this ward – the back ward – for 22 years.

When I think back I realize that my decision to change my ways and co-operate with the staff probably saved my life. At the time I did not think about it this way but now I think about my change as a survival strategy. If I had continued to be rebellious and difficult I would not have survived. If you are in an institution you must follow the rules and obey the staff. That is the only way to survive. I guess I had learned that, even if I wasn't conscious of it at the time. I became friends with the staff and they liked me because I helped out. The work was also good for me. It gave me something to do. In an institution you have all this time on your hands and many people will do almost anything to have something to occupy them. Having nothing to do makes time go very, very slowly. The work also gave me self-respect and the feeling that I was doing something worthwhile.

A visit from my family

I had been in Rome for five years when my father, Belle, Neal and Arlene came to visit me for the first time. It was so good to see them. I had gotten a few letters from Thelma, Marion and Bob, so I had a pretty good idea what was going on. My dad kept moving from one place to another.

We had dinner together at the B-Building. One of the staff went down to the kitchen and brought food for my family. They gave us room, in another part of the building, to be by ourselves so no one would bother us. I was very happy to see them and didn't want them to leave. I wanted them to take me with them. But I knew it wasn't possible. Their visit was a special occasion and it was very hard when they left. Maybe it was their visit that made me want to be more co-operative with the staff. I'm not sure.

In the 22 years I was in H-Building I had a few visits from my family. I also sometimes received letters from them so I could keep up with what was going on in their lives. Later, my sister Marion said she had found it very difficult to come and visit because Rome was such a bad place. But my family never spoke about it when they came and I didn't complain much because I didn't want to spoil the visit. I wanted to have a good time with them while they were there.

Very few visitors came to Rome. Many patients would never get any visits. For others, there would often be many years between visits. Visitors came to the building but they could not come on the ward. The ward was locked. They all were. If someone had visitors they were brought to another part of the building and the patient would be brought down to see them. No one from the outside was allowed on the wards.

Everyday life in the institution

My ordinary day was usually something like the following: I got up at 5.30 in the morning. I was one of the few patients who could tell time and I got up early to help with the morning chores. After I got up, I woke up the working boys,[4] about ten or so of them, and got their routine going. Then I got dressed. A patient helped me dress for the day. After that I went into the day room and supervised the working boys setting the tables for breakfast. The patients who could not move around on their own had to eat at these tables in the day room. The patients ate in two shifts. I sent the boys downstairs to bring up the food. It was brought up in big buckets and was scooped with a ladle onto the plates. There would be cereal, like cornmeal mush, bread and butter, milk and coffee. We didn't get a lot of different choices, we just ate what was there. Once in a while we got prunes for a treat. That was it.

I made sure everyone got fed. I kept my eyes open and made sure the patients who could not eat by themselves got enough to eat. The boys fed those who could not feed themselves. Each of the boys had to feed three or four others at the same time so it would not take too long. If you didn't eat fast enough or didn't want the food, it was thrown in the garbage. About 30 patients would eat in one shift. Each shift was about a half an hour long. I also needed to be fed. One of the boys helped me too. I could not feed myself. I never learned to do that properly. In between shifts I made sure the boys cleaned up and then I sent them downstairs to the dining room to eat their breakfast. All the patients who could get around and feed themselves went downstairs to the dining room.

Everybody who could do a job had a job. The jobs were good because they kept us busy. I did my share and did everything you could imagine. One day a week was bathing day. Everyone got a bath on that day. Staff supervised the working boys who bathed the rest of us. It took several hours. I had a wheelchair I moved with my feet. I got to the clothing room and passed out clean clothes to everyone. In those days people didn't have their own clothes at Rome. Instead, everyone was wearing the white hospital pants and shirts. I picked the clothes off the shelf by size: extra large, large, medium and small. They were all pretty much the same.

On another day we did laundry. All the clothes were piled up in a central location and a truck came and picked them up and brought them to the laundry building where they were washed. I sometimes sorted the laundry but someone else would usually put it away in the clothing room because I had difficulties moving my arms. On other days certain patients were in charge of washing and polishing the floors. There was a big block with straps on it. Old blankets covered the block while it was pushed and pulled across the floor with polish on it.

I also spent my day keeping my eye on the ward. I tried to make sure no one would fight, break windows or make too much noise. If you didn't work, there was not much else to do. There was no TV back then but I turned on the radio so everyone could hear it. There was no programming of any sort. Everyone just sat around in the big day room all day, day after day, week after week, month after month, year after year. The ward always smelled bad. Every 15 or 20 minutes someone would have an accident and one of the other boys would have to clean it up. The patients did most of the work on the ward and the staff supervised.

Staff were usually in charge at lunch and dinner times. Staff set up the tables, got the food and served the meals. The working boys fed everybody like at breakfast. Sometimes people would choke because they had to eat too fast. We ate lunch around eleven o'clock on the ward and those who could go to the dining room ate around noon. That way, they could feed the others before they went down to eat their meals. Dinner was around 4pm on the ward and 5pm downstairs. Right after dinner we started getting everybody ready for bed. The working boys helped the patients who could not undress themselves. Some people got to bed about 7.30pm. I stayed up longer and listened to the radio for a while before I went to bed. Some of us stayed up and listened to the fights on the radio on Friday nights.

Some of the 22 years in this building were good and some were bad. Most of these years the patients were forbidden to go off the ward, except for special occasions, like if a family came for a visit. This changed a little toward the end of my years there. If we wanted to get off the ward for a while we were allowed to go down to the game room. This was our recreation. We got a deck of cards and a box of dominoes and sat around and played for about an hour and a half. There was nothing on the ward to keep us occupied. Not even a deck of cards. Those of the patients who smoked got to leave the ward more often to go down to the game room to smoke. I took up smoking for a little while just to get off the ward. I didn't like it so I quit.

When I was about 48 years old, I got my social security for the first time. Then I started getting my own clothes and things. That made a real difference. I never liked the hospital clothes and I liked having some money to get things for myself, even if it wasn't much.

Trying to better myself

After 22 years in H-Building I decided I wanted to go back to B-Building to try and better myself. The smarter people were in B-Building so I thought I could maybe learn something there. I thought if I really worked hard and tried to learn things my life might change and I would perhaps have my dreams come true. When I think of this now I can see I had bought into the way staff at Rome saw me. I had become convinced I was the problem and if I tried to better myself things would change. And in some sense they did change because I became more co-operative with the staff and worked very hard. I went back there for five years. Then I was offered to go to the new B-Building. I accepted. I moved in 1957 and spent the last 15 years at Rome there. These were some of my best years. For one thing, it was a new building. It did not smell so bad and it had a great big day room with a TV. The living conditions were better but the big difference was the people. I had friends there. They made the real difference.

I did many of the same things as before but here people cared about me and depended on me. Whenever the clothes-room lady was off I would take over the whole thing. In the other buildings I helped out but now I had real responsibilities. It got so I could do most everything. I felt good there because I felt needed and wanted. I was busy and liked my work. I was content for about 15 years and then things began to go backwards. My friends began to leave one by one, for one reason or another. My friends among the staff quit their jobs and left, and my friends among the patients moved to other institutions.

Leaving Rome

In 1973 I decided to call it quits at Rome after 45 years. Things were not going my way. In May or June that year my annual physical came up. I talked to the social worker about moving closer to home. My sister Marion and brother Neal came and I talked to them about moving. Marion came all the way from California, where she was living. They thought it would be a good idea if I could work it out. I kept talking to the social worker. I did most of the talking. They agreed that I could move and decided I should either go to Newark State School, between Rochester and Buffalo, or to Craig State School, near Mt Morris. They finally decided on Craig.

Craig State School

I moved to Craig on 1 November 1973. That was a big day because it was also my birthday. I turned 61 that day. I'll never forget that birthday. I took the trip by ambulance. In those days this was how people were moved from one place to another. They traded one person for me at Rome. It was an even exchange between Craig and Rome – one for one. The first building I stayed in at Craig was the Murphy Building. It was good for a while but it was not a place for me. I got tired of it. If I looked out the windows all I'd see were woods. There was nothing to look at. The Murphy Building was for people who needed close medical supervision. They put me there because I am prone to pneumonia because of my asthma. In the Murphy Building I stayed on the ward all day and had nothing to do. They didn't have any programming and they would not let me help out like I did at Rome. They had a community store and bowling but not much of anything to fill my day up. Nobody had workshops or work to go to then. I watched TV or listened to the tape recorder I owned. I just sat around all day and was terribly bored.

In Craig, like in Rome, all the men were together and all the women were together. We never saw much of each other. They got together for dances and some other things but I never went to them. We didn't even eat in the same dining room.

While I was in Murphy I learned to feed myself. It took me quite a while to learn and I had to take my time to eat. I tried different ways. They had a special spoon they tried with me but I could not use it. They put pillows behind my back to get me closer to the table. I finally got the idea of how to use a spoon and figured out how to hold it without too much trouble. It was amazing to finally learn to feed myself at the age of 62 but it took me so long to eat that the staff did not have time to wait for me. It was much quicker if they fed me so I only fed myself for a short while. It did not help that I did not have many teeth left. In Rome, if we had any problems with our teeth, they were just pulled out, never fixed.

I stayed in the Murphy Building about a year and a half but did not like it, so I decided to get out of there. I talked to my brother Neal. He didn't know what to do. I convinced him to talk to a friend of mine about how to get me out of the Murphy Building. My friend was the head of the speech department and helped me with many things while I was in Craig. He told my brother to write to the director and tell him what building I wanted to move to. Neal wrote to the director and I told him to tell the director that I wanted to move to the Cayuga Building. Cayuga had a more home-like environment. It had nicer furniture. Not just State furniture.

I moved in the spring of 1975. It was a lot better in Cayuga. We used to go for wagon rides. Kind of like a hayride. We put benches on the back of the wagon and about 15 of us would get on and ride all around the grounds. We also saw movies about once a week. They were travel-type movies. I finally got my talking books through a friend of mine who worked at Craig. Once in a while we also went off the grounds to go different places. I got to see plays through the recreation department and I went to Rochester to see some baseball games. I really like baseball and love to go to games. I also went to the community store and bowling. I had a rack where I'd line up the ball and then push the ball hard and it went down the lane to hit the pins down.

I liked Cayuga better than Murphy because I had more to do and because it was more like a home. After I had been in Cayuga for three or four years, they closed the building and I moved down to the Village Green, which was a group of cottage-like buildings. I liked it there. We were 10–12 people in each cottage with two people in each bedroom. I went to work in another building. I packed silverware in plastic. I spent about one and a half to two hours doing this. We got paid by how many pieces we bagged. I used to bring home about two dollars a week. Everything was about the same there as in Cayuga. The guys were still in separate buildings from the ladies.

While I was at Craig I got a motorized wheelchair. It took me a long time to learn how to use it. At first I was always banging into everything but in the end I became really good with it and liked being able to move around on my own for the first time.

They started talking about closing Craig down and I did not want to be caught in the middle. I wanted to decide where I was going to live before someone else decided it for me. I wanted to go into a group home. Many of my friends had moved into group homes. A good friend of mine, who used to work as a speech therapist at Craig, had moved to Syracuse and was working at Syracuse Developmental Center. She told me all about it. It sounded good so I decided to ask for a transfer to Syracuse and thought I would have better chances to go into a group home from there. I applied to move to Syracuse. It took about a year before I moved.

Just about a month before I moved, I got my own room. It was the first and only time in my life I have had a room all to myself. I liked having the privacy. I had applied to go to Syracuse before I knew about the room and I almost changed my mind when I got my own room. But in the end I decided, reluctantly, to go ahead with the move.

Syracuse Developmental Center

I moved into Syracuse Developmental Center (SDC) on 9 March 1982. I was 69 years old. I had my electric wheelchair fixed over after I got there because I wanted to be able to move around on my own. I was on a unit for 20 people and this was the first time I lived on a ward that had both men and women. I shared a bedroom with two other men. The building was fairly new and did not smell too bad. There was a community store and recreational rooms. We would also go off the grounds more than in the other places I had lived in. I enjoyed going out and being part of what was going on in the world outside the institution.

There were some positive things that happened after I moved to Syracuse. One of the most exciting things was to become involved in the resident government at SDC. I became vice-president and was very proud to see us become incorporated. Resident government is for handicapped people to better themselves and speak up for their rights. It was started about ten years before I came to Syracuse by Genevieve Szepanek, one of the residents at SDC. We met about once a week and talked about different subjects. We discussed different problems in the institution and talked about possible ways to solve them. We decided how we would act on the problem and Genevieve wrote to the people concerned. It often took quite a while to get results but in the end we usually got things resolved. We tried to solve problems without making a big deal out of them. We also showed a movie and had a presentation on self-advocacy. Before elections we discussed how to become familiar with the candidates and I voted in the community for the first time.

When I had been at SDC for about two years I could feel myself beginning to slip. I was 70 and felt I was getting old. My health was getting worse. I could no longer use my electric wheelchair and got a push-chair. This made me less independent and more vulnerable to attacks from other residents. I became scared of being hurt and felt I could not defend myself in the violent episodes that occurred regularly. I was fed up with the institution and wanted to be free from these violent surroundings. I wanted to have a home. As an adult I had never lived in a home. My last home was when I was 15 years old, before I moved to Rome, almost 60 years ago. I wanted to have a home before I died. I did not want to die in the institution.

Tom Allen's story continues in Chapter 7 on p.111.

Notes

1 Here Tom uses the term 'crippled' which, at the time, was the most commonly used word to describe physically disabled people.

2 Originally opened in 1894, the Rome State School was first known as the 'Rome State Custodial Asylum for Unteachable Idiots'. In 1903 the name was shortened to the 'Rome State Custodial Asylum', and this is how it was officially known when Tom was first admitted. In 1919, during the period when Tom was living with his family, the name changed again to 'Rome State School'. The name remained unchanged until 1974, when it became the 'Rome Developmental Center'. The Rome Developmental Center closed in 1989. The facility is currently used as a prison.

3 In those days institutional inmates were referred to as 'patients'.

4 In a practice common to most institutions of this era, the Rome State School used higher-functioning inmates as unpaid direct-care 'staff' in the wards housing people with more significant intellectual disabilities or with physical disabilities. These inmates were referred to as 'working boys' or 'working girls'. As Tom's account illustrates, these working boys would actually do many of the daily chores and personal care assigned to the paid attendants for each ward. The free labour not only saved money, it was also one of the ways in which institutions such as Rome tried to cope with the constantly growing pressure of overcrowding.

2

Institutionalization

A Historical Perspective

Jan Walmsley, UK

Today we think it is important that people with intellectual disabilities live in the community rather than in institutions. Institutions are seen as a mistake we made in the past. However, we need to find out more about why people thought institutions were good places for people with intellectual disabilities to live. If we do not understand this then we may make similar mistakes.

There are problems in trying to understand why institutions were thought to be good places for people with intellectual disabilities. We do have some information about institutions that was written when they were seen as the right idea but this information only tells us part of the story and sometimes it is hard to get a clear picture. For example, people with intellectual disabilities did not write about their own experiences until very recently, so we don't have early stories from them. But we do know that there were two very different ideas that led to people thinking that institutions were good places for people to live. One idea was that people with intellectual disabilities were dangerous and caused problems for society. But the other idea which people held at the same time was that people with intellectual disabilities should be looked after and cared for in ways that would enable them to live happy lives.

Not all people with intellectual disabilities went to institutions. And when laws were passed about people with intellectual disabilities they had to be judged to have other characteristics as well as a disability to be 'sent' to an institution; for example, having a child when not married, being guilty of a crime or being cruelly treated by others. Families could decide that their relative would be best cared for in an institution and, at least for some periods of time, families had to pay for their relatives to be there. Sometimes it was difficult for families to gain a place in an institution for their relative. But it was also difficult for people to come out of institutions, even when they or their families wanted them to do so.

People with intellectual disabilities went to institutions for different reasons and we need to be aware that these were not always bad ones. This is not to say that life in institutions was good for the people living there.

This book is about deinstitutionalization. But to understand deinstitutionalization, we need also to appreciate what preceded it – institutionalization. Why did our ancestors choose to place people with intellectual disabilities in institutions? Were they misguided or evil? More misguided and more evil than we are today? To assume this is ahistorical. It is to adopt a simplistic view of the past that sees human life as a progression from darkness to light, an inexorable march of 'progress' in which every age improves on its predecessors. That is clearly untenable. So why, when nowadays we see institutions as such a mistake, did apparently sensible, well-meaning people choose institutions as the answer? I seek to answer these questions here.

In this chapter I explore institutions as a social policy 'solution' to the problem of 'the feeble-minded' in early twentieth-century England, as a means of setting in context the stories in this book. Although England is not entirely representative in its institutionalization practice (for example, unlike in some Scandinavian countries and US states, sterilization was never legalized), the trend to institutionalization there in many respects mirrored similar trends in the English-speaking world (see, for example, Cox *et al.* (1996) on Western Australia, and Trent (1994) on the USA). We know from a number of sources, including some of the testimonies in this book, that, for many of those who lived in them, institutions were unpleasant and restrictive at best, abusive at worst. Yet many intelligent and progressive people of their time (such as playwright George Bernard Shaw and social reformers Sidney and Beatrice Webb) enthusiastically supported the institutionalization of those they called 'the feeble-minded'. How then do we explain why we seem so much more enlightened today, at least as far as people with intellectual disabilities are concerned? The English White Paper *Valuing People* (Department of Health 2001), with its principles of choice, independence, rights and inclusion, could not be further removed from its early twentieth-century equivalent, the 1913 Mental Deficiency Act, which is characterized by segregation, labelling and coercion. We seem to have travelled a long way in just under a century. But has human nature really changed so much? Or are more subtle forces at work, giving the illusion of profound difference when there are considerable elements of continuity?

These are large questions, and in a short chapter I cannot hope to do more than scratch the surface. I address the topic from two angles. The first explores why in the early twentieth century the creation of institutions to house a group called 'the feeble-minded' seemed to contemporaries to be such a good idea. The second considers in more detail the practice of institutions, who got admitted and why, and what became of them once inside. As a number of recent historians have observed, policy is one thing, its implementation often quite another (Armstrong 2002; Read 2004).

For the sake of achievability, the focus is on the first half of the twentieth century, 1900 to 1946. This is the period when the institutionalization of people with intellectual disabilities really got under way. However, before addressing my topic, I want to include some thoughts on the nature of the evidence.

The nature of the evidence

Much of what we know today about institutional life comes from accounts by survivors. Recent trends in intellectual-disability history emphasize a plurality of accounts, and this has contributed to a rich vein of life histories and autobiographies which give us a picture of the institutional experience of patients (Barron

2000; Cooper 1997; Potts and Fido 1991; Rolph 2000; Stuart 2002). This book is adding to those accounts. It is salutary to recall that only just over a decade ago few such accounts had reached print. Our evidence before that date came from institutional records, reports of official inquiries into scandals, the memoirs of former superintendents and staff, and celebratory histories of individual institutions. A very different picture from that given by residents emerges from these sources. Some, such as the Ely Inquiry, do show how impoverished life in hospitals was (HMSO 1969). Others, such as celebratory institutional histories, give a very positive gloss.

Walmsley and Atkinson (2000) published two contrasting accounts of mental deficiency policy in Bedfordshire, an English county, in the post-war period. One, by Cecil French, a former mental welfare officer, subsequently Director of Social Services, told of a shortage of resources and a continual struggle to set up community facilities in the 1950s and 1960s. The other, by a former resident of the local mental handicap hospital, told a totally different story, bringing home the human cost of the policies of the day. But for the early twentieth century such first-hand witness accounts are unobtainable – if only historians a generation ago had taken an interest! We are therefore largely reliant on written sources. Such sources have their own biases and their own constructions of arguments and evidence. This limits what can be deduced reliably. The voices of those subject to the policies, of their families, friends, even staff, are lost, probably forever in most instances. To reconstruct the lives of the people subject to the policies and practices of the early twentieth century we are reliant on what Atkinson and Walmsley (1999) have called 'biographical fragments'; scraps of evidence recorded and stored if they were of enough significance, such as records kept about individuals' certification as 'mental defectives', and their subsequent journeys through the care system.

Moreover, what we read is couched in the arguments and discourses which would carry weight at the time. This can make it hard for us to understand the issues today. The difficulty of interpreting existing discourses has been explored in relation to the sexual abuse of children in the early twentieth century, and is a useful analogy. Brown and Barrett (2002, p.52) discuss the extent to which child prostitution, child sexual abuse and incest were masked in 'vague and euphemistic meaning' in the early twentieth century. There was a tendency to couch arguments for the removal of young girls from their home environments in ways which emphasized their potential to damage or 'contaminate' others, as well as the need for their protection from abuse. The term 'moral danger' conveniently faced both ways – victims of sexual exploitation might both pose a moral danger but also be in moral danger. It was, state Brown and Barrett, a phrase much used by children's charities when removing children from their homes and families, and they quote the following as an example from the files of the Children's Society regarding a nine-year-old:

> The child...is another gutter child and has been brought up to know every charitable person in her neighbourhood and to think all religion cant, she can hardly read and hates school and will do anything to get off being sent to school...worst of all she has been continually sexually assaulted by her own father, while her mother has allowed her to see and hear things which any decent mother would have been careful to keep from the poor little child. The poor little thing has never had a childhood. (quoted in Brown and Barrett 2002, p.51)

There is clear ambivalence here. Was the child a villain or a victim? Similar issues of interpretative difficulty, ambivalence and ambiguity also impact upon our ability to understand the nature of the debates leading to the creation of the segregationist 'solution' to mental deficiency in 1913. Some of these evidential difficulties will be illustrated in the discussion which follows.

The campaign for legislation

The campaign for legislation to deal with the 'problem' of the feeble-minded in Britain reached its apogee in the first decade of the twentieth century. There is consensus amongst historians that people labelled as feeble-minded were seen as responsible for a range of social ills. The fashionable pseudo-science of eugenics led to a concern at the proliferation of the working class, particularly its less respectable members, at the expense of 'better stocks' (Jones 1986, p.18). The poor physical and mental capacity of recruits for the Boer War against South African settlers (1899–1902) and perceptions of a decline in imperial supremacy were prompts for action. The 'feeble-minded' were to blame for these and other social problems and were described as 'the most serious threat to society' (Trent 1994, p.12), partly because, it was argued, they looked like ordinary people, unlike 'idiots' and 'imbeciles'. Tredgold, a contemporary commentator who went on to write the definitive British textbook on 'mental deficiency' (in use until well into the 1970s), listed the ills as abnormally fertile women who gave birth to defective children like themselves, illegitimacy, the spread of venereal disease, criminality, pauperism, and drunkenness. For Tredgold, 'the feeble minded and their relatives form a very considerable proportion, if not the whole, of the social failures and the degenerates of the nation' (quoted in Jones 1986, p.94).

Campaigns by the National Association for the Care of the Feeble Minded (founded 1896) and the Eugenics Education Society (founded 1907) pressed for solutions to the problem of the feeble-minded, based on either segregation or sterilization. They were successful in provoking a Royal Commission which pronounced in 1908. Its conclusions were that there was indeed a case for legislation:

> There are numbers of mentally defective persons whose training is neglected, over whom no sufficient control is exercised, and whose wayward and irresponsible lives are productive of crime and misery, of much injury to themselves and others, and of much continuous expenditure wasteful to the community and to individual families. (HMSO 1908, p.13)

The campaigns for legislation were built on fear, and the predominant arguments were couched in terms of the need to protect society from the menace of the feeble-minded. And yet there was always a subtext of 'care' running through these campaigns. The quote above refers to neglected training. The National Association for the Care of the Feeble Minded included 'care' in its title. Was this mere rhetoric or was there, amongst the scaremongering, a desire to protect individuals as well as society? Mary Dendy, one of the most formidable campaigners for permanent segregation, outlined five main motives for it, the fifth of which was to protect the feeble-minded from society (Jackson 1996, p.161). She, and others, produced numerous examples of children who were exploited and neglected by their parents (Jones 1960, p.13) in support of the Mental Deficiency Bill. Moreover, although recent historians emphasize the coercive nature of the Act (Simonds 1978; Stainton 2000), earlier commentators saw more humane impulses at work. Kathleen Jones, for example, writing in 1960, claimed that the Radnor Commission insisted:

> That the main criterion in certification should be the protection and happiness of the defective rather than 'the purification of the race', and they stressed the possibilities of guardianship as an alternative to permanent segregation. (Jones 1960, p.53)

The Act, which set up a process to identify mental defectives and to manage them, in part through segregation in institutions, was finally passed in 1913. This Act is notorious in British history as one which was coercive and cruel, condemning many to lives inside institutions although, as we shall see below, it was patchy in its application and slow to be implemented.

It is worth pausing here to consider who was subject to the Act. The Act defined four grades of mental deficiency: idiots, imbeciles, feeble-minded persons and moral defectives. Whereas the first three represented different degrees of intellectual disability – we might nowadays call them severe, moderate and mild – moral defectives were different in kind, being people who from an early age displayed 'some permanent mental defect coupled with strong vicious or criminal propensities on which punishment had little or no effect' (Jones 1960, p.67).

The moral defective category made the Act, and the institutions set up under its auspices, a catch-all. The Act could be used to deal with all manner of people, some of whom were unable to function unsupported in society, others of whom were deemed a danger, either because of criminality (boys and men) or because of failure to obey current sexual codes (girls and women). As Abel and Kinder (1942) put it, writing in the context of the USA:

> The subnormals who present a social problem include two groups, of which the first consists of low grade defectives who become a custodial responsibility of the community...and the second is comprised of the high grade subnormals whose institutionalization usually depends upon factors other than subnormality, factors such as emotional instability, social incompetence, and the lack of a requisite economic status in the family or constellation...if the home is broken owing to the death or desertion of a parent...or if the girl, following the urge of adolescent interests, begins to run after the boys or the young men of the neighbourhood, leaving home and refusing to obey her parents, it is very likely that in the course of time it will be considered necessary to remove her from the community by committing her to an institution. (Abel and Kinder 1942, p.105)

However, according to UK law, being deemed a defective was not enough to make a person a 'subject to be dealt with' by the Mental Deficiency Act. The categories of people for whom institutional (or other) provision should be made were, at least in principle, tightly defined. A 'defective' might be sent to an institution or be placed in guardianship if his or her parents petitioned for it or if he or she was neglected, abandoned, cruelly treated and without visible means of support; guilty of a criminal offence; in prison, reformatory, industrial school, lunatic asylum or inebriate reformatory; a habitual drunkard; incapable of receiving benefit from attendance at a special school or a woman pregnant with, or bearing, an illegitimate child whilst in receipt of poor relief. Therefore, given this list, there was no carte blanche for people, even if certified 'defective', to be detained in institutions, with certain notable exceptions, particularly people convicted of a criminal offence or poor women bearing illegitimate children. The role of families was critical, so that one historian claims that 'families, at least in the early days of mental deficiency asylums, were influential in drawing up the criteria for defining admission to asylum' (Stuart 2002, p.10).

The extent to which institutions, as envisaged under this Act, were seen as protective and rehabilitative, as opposed to coercive and designed to restrain people's liberty, is debatable. I would argue that because of the 'moral defective' category, there can be no doubt that prevention of reproduction and criminality was always a paramount consideration.

However, institutions also housed people who were genuinely unable to function autonomously. There was always a rhetoric of protection. A textbook for people charged with implementation of the Act tried to define 'neglect', one of the most commonly cited reasons for institutionalization:

> A defective may be deemed to be neglected if the person or persons who have a duty to care for him do not fulfil this duty...lack of protection from moral danger or exposure to physical or moral dangers have been regarded as proof of neglect...in the case of a girl, that the father had been convicted of an offence under the Criminal Law Amendment Act in respect to any of his daughters. (Shrubsall and Williams 1932, pp.255–256)

Similarly, 'cruelly treated' is discussed: 'An imbecile child kept most of the day chained up to a dog kennel while the parents were out at work' is cited as a case of a person being 'cruelly treated' (Shrubsall and Williams 1932, p.257). In a period when community facilities were rudimentary, arguably some people saw institutions as protective.

Pains were also taken to emphasize that institutions were viewed not as a home for life but as a means of restoring people to the community:

> The modern aim is gradually to restore such a person to the community provided that adequate steps can be taken to avoid his falling into misconduct or becoming a parent. (Shrubsall and Williams 1932, p.184)

This emphasis echoes the vision of the Wood Committee, which reported in 1929, of the institution not as a 'stagnant pool, but...a flowing lake, always taking in and always sending out' (HMSO 1929, p.71).

Later historians have also defended the Act. Writing of the work of the Wood Committee in the 1920s, Jones comments:

> The distinction between the patient in hospital and the patient under voluntary supervision had nothing to do with his scholastic ability. It depended entirely on whether he was capable of leading a normal life under reasonably sheltered conditions without being exploited himself or causing difficulty in his environment. Those who were anti social or in moral danger (such as alcoholics or over sexed young women) would continue to need institutional care; but the quiet stable kind of defective, even with a comparatively low intelligence, might be discharged to the care of a suitable social worker. (Jones 1960, p.85)

At a time when almost all provision for poor, disabled or mentally ill people was punitive and regimented, Jones regarded institutionalization as motivated by a desire to help and protect, as well as curb and control. But what of the reality?

Institutional practice: what do we know?

We have seen that legislation had within it some reformist zeal, alongside the ever-present social control motive. In principle, people could move into and out of the institution, having been rescued from moral danger, neglect or ill-treatment. Did this actually happen?

There is certainly evidence that some people were institutionalized to protect them, though often this was couched in obscure language. 'Dora', for example, was examined for mental deficiency in 1915. She had been 'without visible means of support' after being discharged from domestic service for 'behaving immorally with farm hands'. Her stepfather, when questioned, said he would not receive her back as she had accused him of 'attempting immoral conduct with her' (Bedfordshire County Record Office Mental Deficiency Papers vol. 3, 1915). Dora was subsequently institutionalized. As Atkinson and Walmsley (1999, p.207) comment: 'today she might well be categorised as an abused woman, that is her biography would be recast to present her as a "victim" rather than as feeble minded.'

However, there are clear indications that sexual control was paramount, particularly early in the period of the Mental Deficiency Act, when institutional places were at a premium. My study of case records in the Bedford Record Office 1916–1918 (Walmsley 2000) shows that of the 35 people before the county's Mental Deficiency Committee in those years, 19 were sent to institutions. Of these, four were male, three of whom were under the age of 18. All were detained after falling into petty crime. Of the 15 women who were institutionalized, 11 were described as displaying inappropriate sexual behaviour – the four others were clearly victims of neglect due to the inability or unwillingness of family to care for them.

Drawing on work by Cox (1996) and Thomson (1998), as well as my own documentary research, I concluded that poverty, moral worth, respectability or otherwise of the family and employability of the person were factors influencing decisions to institutionalize young women. People who were seriously mentally impaired, on the other hand, were unlikely to acquire an institutional place unless their families were completely unable to care for them (Walmsley 2000). Women who could be placed in domestic service were far more likely to be subsequently released from institutional care on licence. As Rolph has observed, such employment could supply the surveillance over people's lives that was deemed necessary (Rolph 2000). Thomson's analysis of London's records also suggests that men were likely to spend far less time in institutional care than women, and to be institutionalized at an earlier age (Thomson 1998).

We have very little direct knowledge from inmates themselves. One rare example is a letter to the Clerk to the Mental Deficiency Committee in Bedfordshire from a woman called Ruth Gammon, dating from 1943. It is the first example I have found of what we now term self-advocacy, even using the phrase Ken Simons used for the title of his study of self-advocacy: 'sticking up for yourself' (Simons 1992).

> Dear Madame or Sir,
>
> I wonder if you would in any way do me a great favour. All I want to ask you is could you by any means help me to get discharge from the care and control. As this is my 21 years I done under your care and control. I am 36 years old. I done 15 years and six months at Stoke Park and 12 months at Bromham House. But I am at Springfield House in service for four years and four months. This is the first time I have written to you. Nothing like sticking up for yourself.
>
> But I must thank you for putting me under your care and control in the first place. I don't know where I would have been. But now I am able to look after myself. (Bedfordshire County Record Office Joint Board Papers 1943)

The committee agreed to release her from the terms of the Act, after a positive report from the hospital – 'good moral character' – and a favourable reference to a mother and sister living locally.

What do we make of the final sentence? She thanks the committee for putting her under 'care and control'. Is this merely a rhetorical flourish to please the powerful men who held her fate in their hands? Or did she mean it?

This example dates from war time, when staff shortages made discharge of those who were able highly desirable. However, there is plenty of evidence that people were detained beyond the period when they might have been considered to be rehabilitated. Part of the reason for this was in the economics of institutions which relied on patient labour. Bromham House in Bedfordshire was described as an asset which 'can form a workshop wherein much useful work can be effected for the local authority' (sic) (Bromham House Annual Report 1943). There was open acknowledgement that patients contributed hugely to the running of institutions: 'It is worthy of note to what extent these helpless ones are mothered by those who are only usually mixed with their own class' (Bedfordshire Joint Board Papers 1939). Robert McKenzie, a patient of Lennox Castle Hospital in Scotland from 1947 to 1999, recalled the work he had done, soon after the war:

> I used to help all the nurses every night. I got the laundry bags all ready for the wee ones to change at night. Tied the laundry and put it outside for the motors to take away. I shifted the coal in the boiler house, heavy work. Aye, I looked after somebody as well. I used to take the wee boy out for a walk... I'd feed all the wee ones that couldn't hold a spoon. I'd take the plates into the day hall and feed the ones that were handicapped. (McKenzie 2002)

There were sewing rooms and mat-making rooms, farms and laundries, shoe-repair workshops and carpentry, engineering and tailoring – and care for less able patients – all of which were operated by patient labour, virtually unremunerated; cigarette or sweet allowances were the commonest form of payment (Bromham House Annual Report 1939). Some parents argued for the release of their sons and daughters from institutions on the grounds that they were being kept for their economic worth. For example, the family of Abel John Davies, who absconded from Bromham Hospital in 1940, sheltered him and accused the hospital authorities of hanging on to him to make money out of him (Bedfordshire Joint Board Papers 1940). There are also indications that some privately run institutions kept hold of the more able patients, despite the wishes of the local authority which was obliged to pay for the place.

Once deinstitutionalization of the more able patients got under way in the 1950s, the cost implications began to be recognized:

> The policy of discharging suitable patients on licence whenever possible has continued with perhaps added impetus recently, depriving the hospital of

> many willing hands capable of useful employment. Tasks undertaken by patients must now be undertaken by staff, and it has become necessary to augment the establishment. (Bedford Group of Hospitals 1958, p.15)

A further key question about institutions is the degree to which they were supported by families. The simplistic view of the past sees children being wrenched from their loving families to be 'put away'. This is by no means the whole picture. There has been some debate over whether parents were or were not in favour of their sons or daughters entering into and, more significantly, remaining in institutions (Thomson 1998). The picture is complicated by economic factors. In the UK, families had to pay towards the costs of institutional care on a sliding scale according to income (this ended in 1946 with the inception of the National Health Service), and much of the correspondence in the files of mental deficiency committees relates to chasing up payment arrears. Not only did families lose their relatives, they also had to pay. The picture is genuinely mixed. Some families did petition for a place, but often to no avail. Certainly in the 1920s and later, parents were unlikely to be successful in requesting institutional care for their sons or daughters, unless there were other factors such as sexual misconduct or criminal behaviour, making it seem a desirable option. Records of mental deficiency committees in Bedfordshire and Northamptonshire, two English counties, include instances of families asking for an institutional place and being turned down. One, dating from 1938, is mentioned in a letter from the Bedfordshire Clerk to the parents:

> Up to the present time, owing partly to the great difficulty being experienced in obtaining the necessary nursing staff, cases such as that of your daughter have not been admitted to the colony. (Bedfordshire Mental Deficiency Committee Letters 10/8/38)

This is by no means an isolated example. Parents, in part because they had no community supports, often did want their children taken off their hands. However, some families fought hard against the system which took away their sons and daughters. It required incredible persistence in negotiating with the bureaucracy of the Act. May Bellamy's aunt displayed great energy in fighting for her niece to be allowed out on leave from Bromham Hospital in 1944. She was told that May was: 'Obstinate, truculent, foul mouthed and grossly lacking in moral sense' (Bedfordshire and Northamptonshire Joint Board Papers 1944). The aunt was undeterred, continued to write and engaged a solicitor to make the case. She was not successful.

Ernest Bateman's sister and brother wrote three or four times every year for five years (at least) in the 1940s to request leave of absence for him. Each time, the case had to be referred to the medical superintendent, and then a home visit was conducted to establish whether the home was suitable. Ernest's sister and brother also challenged the practice of censoring Ernest's mail. They were told:

> All letters to or from a patient may be read by the Superintendent and if the contents are objectionable the letter need not be forwarded or delivered. No letters are censored. (Bedfordshire and Northamptonshire Joint Hospital Board Papers 14/i)

Other families were less enthusiastic – or perhaps had fewer resources. There are instances of the Bedfordshire and Northamptonshire Joint Hospital Board writing to parents suggesting they take their relative home on leave of absence in the 1930s, and getting the reply that they could not afford the travel (patients had to be escorted home), or there was no space and no means to support the person. Just occasionally grants were made to families to come to Bromham in order to collect their relative or to visit, again in the 1930s (Bedfordshire Mental Deficiency Papers).

Parents and families were often complicit in the act of committing their offspring to institutions. There is some evidence that they were less enthusiastic when they realized they were not coming out!

There seems little doubt that, whether or not the reasons for removing a person to an institution were motivated by humanitarian objectives, institutions became an end in themselves, sustaining their own reasons for existence, and resisting criticism and change. Michael McFadden, a nurse employed at Lennox Castle Hospital in Scotland, reflected that:

> When Lennox Castle opened in '36 it was heralded as the best example of care for the mentally deficient in Britain. People came from all over to see it...so everyone thought that was the best thing... Everybody thought 'we are providing the best care that can be provided.' It's a question of evolution; time has moved. I think there's no doubt that it was the best example of care available, but instead of maybe moving forward and maybe embracing new ideas as they came, I think the hospital probably did – and I would be part of it – stagnate somewhat in the 50s, 60s and 70s. (McFadden 2002)

There was undoubtedly stagnation in patient careers also. Although technically patients' detention had to be reviewed after one year, and thenceforward at five-yearly intervals, in effect medical superintendents had the final say over release, and frequently they took a judgemental line (the description of May Bellamy quoted above was far from unique) and resisted arguments for ending the placement. There was considerable complacency too. In a year (1943) when there had been 70 instances of people absconding from his hospital, the medical superintendent of Bromham Hospital wrote of the contentment of patients, and the training they were receiving (Bromham House Annual Report 1943).

Other than Ruth Gammon's testimony quoted earlier in this chapter and records of escapes, there is very little direct testimony from residents from the years before the National Health Service. The evidence is certainly mixed in regard to the volition of families, some of whom seemed quite eager to have their offspring admitted to institutions, others less so. It seems they had more difficulty extracting people once they were in. Institutions, guided by the professional judgement of those who ran them, had a way of becoming an end in themselves rather than a means to an end – rehabilitation and discharge – and given the economic contribution both in terms of labour and in terms of contributions families made to maintenance that is perhaps unsurprising. The National Council for Civil Liberties campaign of the 1950s highlighted the infringements of human rights that had become the norm, and the lack of safeguards against what could very easily be a life sentence (Stainton 2000).

Conclusion

Institutional care for people with intellectual disabilities has rightly had a bad press. Nevertheless, it remains the case that there are people in every society for whom life unsupported by others is impossible. For much of the twentieth century this support was provided for people with intellectual disabilities either by their families or in institutions. One of my intentions in writing this chapter has been to provoke a more nuanced consideration of why institutions gained such a hold. To dismiss two or three generations out of hand as purely evil and coercive is an oversimplification. There is no defending what institutions became with poor funding and low aspirations. However, there is, I believe, a case for recognizing that every generation has to find its own solutions to the challenge presented by adults unable to care for themselves, and that some genuinely believed that institutions were indeed preferable to the alternative – neglect.

During 2005 the last mental handicap hospitals in England will finally close. This is rightly seen as a historic achievement. This does not, however, mean that institutions are dead and gone. Anyone who knows the realities of life for people with intellectual disabilities will also know that plenty of institutions remain; in the UK these are frequently run under the auspices of the voluntary sector. They will also know that institutional practices can be found in community facilities, large and small. To focus exclusively on institutions as the evil to be fought could conceivably distract attention from the real evils which are inhumane treatment, neglect and denial of rights. It is important to place the era of institutional care, now coming to a close, in perspective, and to recognize that the story is a more complex one than is usually acknowledged.

There is much still to discover about institutional life and the dynamics behind the institutional solution in the twentieth century. If I have only aroused in readers the desire to know more, I will feel the effort to write this chapter has been worthwhile.

References

Abel, T. and Kinder, E.F. (1942) *The Subnormal Adolescent Girl.* New York: Columbia University Press.

Armstrong, F. (2002) 'The historical development of special education: Humanitarian rationality or "wild profusion of tangled events".' *History of Education 31*, 5, 437–56.

Atkinson, D. and Walmsley, J. (1999) 'Using autobiographical approaches with people with learning disabilities.' *Disability and Society 14*, 2, 203–217.

Barron, D. (2000) 'From community to institution and back again.' In L. Brigham, D. Atkinson, M. Jackson, S. Rolph and J. Walmsley (eds) *Crossing Boundaries: Change and Continuity in the History of Learning Disability.* Kidderminster: BILD.

Bedford Group Hospital Management Committee (1958) *Bedford Group of Hospitals Survey 1948–1958.* London: North West Metropolitan Regional Health Authority.

Brown, A. and Barrett, D. (2002) *Knowledge of Evil: Child Prostitution and Child Sexual Abuse in Twentieth Century England.* London: Wilan Publishing.

Cooper, M. (1997) 'Mabel Cooper's life story.' In D. Atkinson, M. Jackson and J. Walmsley (eds) *Forgotten Lives.* Kidderminster: BILD.

Cox, E., Fox, C., Brogan, M. and Lee, M. (1996) *Under Blue Skies: The Social Construction of Intellectual Disability in Western Australia.* Perth: Edith Cowan University, Centre for Disability Research and Development.

Cox, P. (1996) 'Girls, deficiency and delinquency.' In D. Wright and A. Rigby (eds) *From Idiocy to Mental Deficiency: Historical Perspectives on People with Learning Disabilities.* London: Routledge.

Department of Health (2001) *Valuing People: A New Strategy for Learning Disability for the 21st Century.* London: HMSO.

HMSO (1908) *Royal Commission on the Care and Control of the Feeble Minded, Report* (the Radnor Commission). London: HMSO.

HMSO (1929) *Mental Deficiency Committee* (the Wood Report). London: HMSO.

HMSO (1969) *Report of the Committee of Inquiry into Allegations of Ill Treatment of Patients and Other Irregularities at Ely Hospital Cardiff* (Cmnd 3975). London: HMSO.

Jackson, M. (1996) 'Institutional provision for the feeble minded. Sandlebridge and the scientific morality of permanent care.' In D. Wright and A. Rigby (eds) *From Idiocy to Mental Deficiency: Historical Perspectives on People with Learning Disabilities.* London: Routledge.

Jones, G. (1986) *Social Hygiene in Twentieth Century Britain.* London: Croom Helm.

Jones, K. (1960) *Mental Health and Social Policy, 1854–1959.* London: Routledge and Kegan Paul.

McFadden, M. (2002) Testimony from M. McFadden and R. McKenzie. In Lennox Castle Exhibition: The Human History of an Institution (2002).

McKenzie, R. (2002) Testimony from M. McFadden and R. McKenzie. In Lennox Castle Exhibition: The Human History of an Institution (2002).

Potts, M. and Fido, R. (1991) *A Fit Person to be Removed.* Plymouth: Northcote House.

Read, J. (2004) 'Fit for what? Special education in London 1890–1914.' *History of Education 33*, 3, 283–98.

Rolph, S. (2000) 'The History of Community Care for People with Learning Difficulties in Norfolk 1913–1970: The Story of Two Hostels.' Unpublished PhD Thesis. Open University: Milton Keynes.

Shrubsall, F. and Williams, A. (1932) *Mental Deficiency Practice.* London: University of London Press.

Simonds, H. (1978) 'Explaining social policy: The English Mental Deficiency Act of 1913.' *Journal of Social History 11*, 387–403.

Simons, K. (1992) *'Sticking up for Yourself': Self Advocacy and People with Learning Difficulties.* London/York: Joseph Rowntree Foundation.

Stainton, T. (2000) 'Equal citizens? The discourse of liberty and rights in the history of learning disabilities.' In L. Brigham, D. Atkinson, M. Jackson, S. Rolph and J. Walmsley (eds) *Crossing Boundaries: Change and Continuity in the History of Learning Disability* pp.87–102. Kidderminster: BILD.

Stuart, M. (2002) *Not Quite Sisters.* Kidderminster: BILD.

Thomson, M. (1998) *The Problem of Mental Deficiency: Eugenics, Democracy and Social Policy in Britain c. 1870–1959.* Oxford: Clarendon Press.

Trent, J. Jr. (1994) *Inventing the Feeble Mind: A History of Mental Retardation in the United States.* Berkeley, CA: University of California Press.

Walmsley, J. (2000) 'Women and the Mental Deficiency Act of 1913: Citizenship, sexuality and regulation.' *British Journal of Learning Disabilities 28*, 2, 65–70.

Walmsley, J. and Atkinson, D. (2000) 'Oral history and the history of learning disability.' In J. Bornat, R. Perks, P. Thompson and J. Walmsley (eds) *Oral History, Health and Welfare.* London: Routledge.

Archive sources

Bedfordshire and Northamptonshire Joint Board (Bromham Hospital) Papers

Bedfordshire County Record Office Mental Deficiency Papers

Bedfordshire Joint Board Papers

Bedfordshire Mental Deficiency Committee Letters

Bedfordshire Mental Deficiency Committee Papers

Bromham House Annual Report

3

Containing Uncontainable Women

Kelley Johnson, Australia

Brigid Anderson and Jane King lived in a locked unit in a large institution for people with intellectual disabilities in Australia called Hilltop. I spent 20 months with them and with the other women in their unit as their institution closed. They were confined to a locked unit because they were labelled as having challenging behaviours. Brigid had lived all her life in institutions; she sometimes attacked other women and staff, banged her head on the walls and stripped off her clothes. Jane had been sexually abused by the men in her family from when she was a small child. She had lived at different times in the community and in institutions. She lived in the locked unit because she had attacked a staff member with a knife. Jane was sometimes very angry and attacked staff in the unit. She also liked sex and staff were concerned that she would have sex with people in order to get cigarettes and alcohol.

When the institution was closing, people living there were asked where they would like to live. Brigid could not speak but her advocate said that she should have a chance to live in the community. Jane wanted very much to return to the community where she had lived before. Her advocate believed that she should not do so, and she chose to live in a house on the grounds of another institution.

However, in the end both women were sent to live in other large institutions.

This happened for a number of reasons: staff at the institution had strong views about the women and where they should live, and their voices were important. Neither woman had a strong advocate or family member who could support her move into the community. Luck had something to do with it too. Brigid almost went to live in the community but the decision-maker was persuaded not to allow it after a lunch meeting with a staff member. Jane's file was lost and she did not get as much consideration about where she might live as other people. People saw institutions as strong places that could hold people who were difficult to be with. They thought that the community would not be able to do this. Locking these women away in an institution meant that people did not have to try and understand their pain and anger.

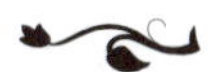

Kelley writes: The stories of the two women whose lives are described in this chapter, Brigid Anderson and Jane King, were collected from a range of different sources. Jane was able to tell me something of her story, though mostly in terms of the things she wanted or had enjoyed. Brigid was not able to use spoken language. I spent 20 months as a participant observer with them and 19 other women in the locked unit within a large institution where they lived. During this time the institution closed. I also gathered information from discussions with staff at the institution and from the records that were kept at the institution about each of them. I then wrote the stories based on this information.

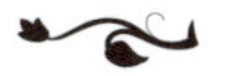

In spite of the movement across many different countries to close total institutions for people with intellectual disabilities, and continuing research evidence that supports community living as a better option than congregate care (Emerson and Hatton 1996; Kim, Larsen and Lakin 2001; Young *et al.* 1998), some people continue to find it extremely difficult to find a place in the community. Why is this so? Arguments are advanced in the literature that the people who are left in the institutions are those who are most difficult to 'manage' in the community, either because of the degree of support they require or because of challenging behaviour (Day 1994; Dosen 1994; Johnson 1998). But what do these things mean in practice for individuals? How are these individuals perceived by those around them? And what other factors are involved in deciding that a person should continue to live within an institution?

This chapter explores these questions by describing the lives of Brigid Anderson and Jane King, two women who lived in a locked unit within an institution called Hilltop, in Australia. They were both young women with much of their lives in front of them. When the institution in which they lived closed, approximately half of the women who had lived there went to live in the community. Neither of these two women did. After consultation they were moved to other total institutions in the state. In this chapter I will describe the lives the women led in the locked unit and then examine why this decision was made.

Brigid Anderson

> Brigid is a slight woman who is under five feet tall. She has short sparse brown hair (which she pulls out), a round elfish face and brilliant blue eyes.
>
> In common with most of the women in the locked unit, her two front teeth have been removed to prevent her from biting herself or other people. Brigid has a wicked chuckle and shouts and screams loudly. She does not speak or use any sign language. She is always alert to movement around the unit and watches the other women carefully. Brigid has no family [and] no friends... Brigid is one of the youngest women living in the unit. (Johnson 1998, p.24)

Brigid was 26 years old when I met her and had spent her whole life in an institution. She had been in the locked unit for eight years. She was born to a very young woman who placed her immediately in the care of nuns. Brigid stayed with the nuns for the first 12 months of her life before being moved to a large institution for people with intellectual disabilities. She stayed in the first institution for two years before being moved to Hilltop where I met her. Staff commented that Brigid was tiny as a child and was often carried around all day by staff members as they did their work. As she grew older she became aggressive to other children and her behaviour was regarded as difficult to manage by staff. She was moved to a locked unit when she was 18 years old.

As a child she had enjoyed going to school, but when she left there was nothing for her to do. She spent all of her days in a large locked room with 20 other women. Staff did not take her outside the unit on walks or excursions, as when they did she sat down and refused to return to the unit.

My first encounter with Brigid was by hearsay. She was nicknamed 'the devil's child' and older staff commented that Satan had entered her through a scar on her body. Her reputation for hair pulling, biting and smearing faeces was fearsome. Some staff refused to work in the unit because of her behaviour. Others who had worked with her spoke of her with warmth and pity. One staff member commented that she 'reminds me of my little girl'.

When I first met her, Brigid was sitting on a sofa in the day room. She was rapidly and efficiently stripping off her clothes which she hurled across the room. Once naked she would sit on the couch surveying the room and its occupants. Staff used a number of often bizarre strategies to clothe her. These included dressing her again, removing her clothes once she had taken them off and putting them on a high shelf, and donning Brigid's clothes themselves. There was no consistency in staff response to her behaviour and she greeted all strategies with laughter, a shout of rage or physical resistance.

Brigid's behaviour was unpredictable. Sometimes she would touch her genitals repeatedly. Sometimes she would laugh uproariously at something of which only she was aware. At other times she would bang her head violently against the walls or the table. She would attack other women without warning. Usually this involved seizing the other woman by the hair and pulling her head down. Sometimes she attempted to bite people, and staff and other women in the unit were very wary of her. She could also be affectionate and loving. She would blow kisses to staff in the unit and enjoyed games of jumping high and peek-a-boo. But these activities could quickly change into more aggressive behaviour. She would sometimes cuddle up on the couch with a staff member, who would stroke her and hold her close.

Brigid had a territory within the unit. She would run the full length of the day room, slamming the door to the bathroom if for some reason it was unlocked and then hurl herself on to a couch. She would move around the room from couch to couch.

During the closure of the institution there was a consultation about the future of each resident with family, advocates, staff and the person him- or herself. Brigid was not able to be an active participant in the consultation, but a former staff member advocated strongly that she be able to go into the community. When the final decisions were made about relocation, there was some support from a community case manager that she be given a chance. In fact, the decision seemed to have been made that she would go to a house in a country town. However, over lunch the manager of the locked unit persuaded the community case manager not to include Brigid in the community because of her challenging behaviour. Because she had no family near whom she could live or who could advocate for her, Brigid's relocation was finally determined by where there was an empty bed. She was relocated to a country institution. She remained at the institution in the country for some years but now lives in supported accommodation in a country town.

Jane King

Jane was a young woman in her early thirties with brown hair and a round face. She was one of the few women in the locked unit to have a room of her own and she spent a lot of time there, sitting on the bed and watching television. The room was tiny with a floor that sloped down at one side. The walls were corrugated iron. But it was her own place. Jane had spent much of her childhood in and out of care. She had lived with her family for some time but had been sexually abused by both her father and her brothers. She had then been taken into State care and had experienced both institutional living and foster care. She had also lived with an aunt for some time. In adulthood this pattern continued. Jane had lived relatively independently in the community for varying lengths of time. She had committed some minor offences, including thieving a handbag from a passer-by, but had not been convicted of any crimes. She enjoyed partying and an active sexual life. This led to her gaining a reputation among staff as being 'promiscuous', and her advocate commented that she had traded sex for cigarettes and alcohol. She had spent some time in supported accommodation but had been sent to the institution because her presence 'caused trouble' among the men living in the accommodation. She had a reputation for anger and aggression in many of the services which she had used. For some time she lived in a house on the grounds of Hilltop but she attacked a staff member with a knife and was sent to live in the locked unit. She had been there for two years.

She continued to have episodes of anger, was sent for anger-management therapy, saw a psychiatrist intermittently and at one stage was sent to a psychiatric hospital for treatment. She returned from hospital with a report which said that her impulsive anger was due solely to her intellectual disability and that she should remain in institutional care. Efforts were made by staff in the unit to identify when Jane was becoming frustrated or angry. They then isolated her and treated the anger either by telling her to 'throw teddy' (a teddy bear) or by medication.

Jane was an extroverted woman who clearly enjoyed partying and sex. She was the only woman in the unit with a boyfriend. However, he was banned because of staff fears that he might have HIV/AIDS. Her family was also banned from visits because of continuing sexual abuse.

There can be little doubt that Jane was extremely frustrated in the locked unit. She spent a lot of time smoking cigarettes, watching television and talking with staff. She had no friendships among the other women in the unit. She wanted to leave the unit and was told by the unit manager that this could only happen if she could control her anger for three months. This seemed an impossible demand given the stressful nature of unit life. Jane had not received any counselling for the sexual abuse she had experienced as both a child and an adult, nor was this taken into account in assessments of her anger. Unlike most of the other women in the unit, Jane had a guardian who could make decisions about her accommodation, health and other areas of her life.

When Jane learned the institution was closing she was very excited. She hoped that this would enable her to move again to the community, be with her friends (who did not visit her in the institution) and live a more independent life. She made promises to 'be a good girl' and talked about the parties she would go to when she left the institution. During the consultation her first preference had been for a house in the community. However, her guardian vetoed this possibility and Jane was urged to choose a house in the grounds of another institution. The following note from my field notes describes what happened when the final decision was made as to Jane's future living arrangements.

> I arrived in the room where Jane's preferences were being considered half way through the afternoon. Her first preference was for a house on the grounds at Rochester [an institution for people with intellectual disabilities]. It was hot and the panel members (who made the decisions) looked exhausted and frustrated both by the work done, and that which remained.
>
> They had spent the day attempting to juggle more than forty people who wanted a house on the grounds at Rochester with the twenty-one places available. ... When I looked at the whiteboard with its names and houses I realised that Jane's name was not there. I pointed this out to the panel chairperson.
>
> The names were checked and concern was expressed by the panel members at the omission, particularly because the allocation to houses was now almost set. A member of the relocation panel was sent to look for Jane's

> file. He went reluctantly and returned to state that Jane had already been matched to a unit in another institution. He said that this solved the problem of having to consider her for a match with a house on the grounds at Rochester. One of the...[panel members] stated strongly that this was unfair and that Jane should be considered for matching. ... [Her] file was large as the CCOR[1] convenor thought Jane's best hope for a positive matching was to provide all the information available. Instead the panel saw the size of the file and someone said 'God look at this, not this one.' Bits of the file were read out which described Jane's aggressive behaviour. Within three minutes the panel had decided that she should not be matched to a house on the grounds. Jane was matched to a unit in a city institution. (Johnson 1998, pp.117–8)

Jane is still living in a locked unit within an institution.

Reflections

Both of these young women failed the test they were given when their institution closed. They were judged not to be able to live in the community. The explicit reasons given for this were those of duty of care to the woman with a disability and danger to the community. However, there was also a more pragmatic reason. There were only sufficient resources to fund half the residents in supported accommodation in the community. The rest had to go to other institutions. The cards were stacked.

There is no doubt that, while Jane and Brigid had very different life experiences and disabilities, they were both difficult women to be with. However, the description of the closure processes suggests that factors other than their need for high support or their perceived dangerousness or challenging behaviour were important in the decision that they should stay in an institution.

Family and advocates

Neither of these women had a strong advocate who supported her movement to the community. Brigid's advocate, a former staff member, was keen for her to have a chance to live outside an institution. However, she did not see Brigid often and was not seen as someone with whom Brigid would have continuing contact. Consequently, her views were not taken very seriously by the people undertaking the consultation. Jane had a formal guardian who believed that she was both sexually vulnerable and dangerous. He was opposed to her leaving the institution although supportive of her living in a house on the grounds of another institution. He did not have a strong relationship with Jane but relied heavily on the files and staff input for his knowledge.

Staff views

In both of these women's cases, staff views about them were extremely important. It was almost certain that Brigid would have gone to a house in the country had the panel member not had lunch with her unit manager. The unit manager was generally a fair woman but was concerned about Brigid's behaviour and there was no mitigating voice from her advocate to be heard. Nor was Brigid known to the panel member. In Jane's case, the staff member who spoke negatively about her did not know her very well, except by reputation, but his voice was one of authority in a group of panel members who had never met Jane and knew little of her background. In Jane's case, had the unit manager been consulted a different picture may have emerged.

Neglected histories

The files that were given to people making decisions about community living were voluminous about both these women. They documented their challenging behaviour, their family connections (or lack thereof) and told something of their preferences. However, they did not provide information that might have helped to explain the women's behaviour or to place it in a context. Jane had been sexually abused from childhood by all the men in her family. She had not received counselling for this nor was it taken into account in considering her behaviour or her placement. Her frustration at living in a locked room with 20 other women, almost none of whom offered any companionship to her, was not considered either. Rather, it was seen as her responsibility to 'prove' that she could be 'a good girl' and earn a place in the community. The effects of long-term institutional life on Brigid were not taken into account nor were the possible traumatic long-term effects of her rejection by her mother (Sinason 1992). Both women were judged on their present behaviours; they were women with no history.

Chance

Just as chance had played its role in leading to the admission of these women to an institution, so it played a role in deciding their fates when the institution closed. If the panel member had not met the unit manager over lunch, Brigid would have gone to the community. If Jane's file had not been misplaced she may have got a better hearing in the panel. If... Regardless of their disability and 'challenging behaviour', judgements were made about these women which owed a considerable amount to chance occurrences on the day decisions were made.

Gender issues

Neither of these women fulfilled the societal stereotypes of being a woman. They were angry, aggressive and loud. This was enough to make it difficult for them to live in the community. Yet, paradoxically, Jane was in part confined to the institution because of her sexuality as a woman. Sexual promiscuity was seen as evidence of vulnerability and she was confined with no real attempt at providing any education which could lead to her having a safe sexual life. These women were caught in judgements which institutionalized them in part because they did not match stereotypes of being women and in part because of their gender.

The role of institutions

Institutions were seen as 'bad' by all those involved in the deinstitutionalization of Hilltop. They were perceived as offering a poor quality of life, segregating people and denying their rights. The process of judgement about who should continue to reside in an institution also revealed that they were seen as containing people who were 'bad'. It was only those who were so categorized in terms of dangerousness or 'challenging behaviour' or 'high support needs' who were to remain in institutional 'care'. The institution was perceived to be the place that was both a physical container for people and one which could also hold their propensities for disruption and 'uncontainability'. It was seen as invulnerable to their behaviour. Brigid and Jane were seen to be women who belonged in such a place. In this scenario the community was perceived to be a 'good' place which could include those people who had maintained relationships with families, who were quiet and submissive and who did not require high support. In contrast to the institution, the community was viewed as 'vulnerable', unable to contain these women.

Lack of attachment

Within all of us there are both creative and destructive aspects. In the community it is fundamental to our well-being that we hold each other emotionally, parents with children and families with each other (Bion 1991; Bion 1993). Brigid and Jane had not had the emotional holding as children that made it easy for people to hold them in this way as adults. They had been abandoned or betrayed by their families. Their lives had been filled with abuse, deprivation and isolation. Their feelings of anger, frustration, fear and despair (shown in their behaviours) made it difficult for anyone to help them bear the pain. As a result, they were held within the physical walls of the institution which contained what were seen as their destructive behaviours. Physical walls were a substitute for emotional containment. The continued institutionalization of these women absolved people from the need to understand or bear some of the pain and anger that they felt.

Conclusion

I worked closely with Brigid and Jane over an extended period of time. I am not arguing in this chapter that they were easy to get along with or that they did not have disabilities and problems. However, in the closure of the institution decisions were made which did not really focus on these women as individuals. Rather, these decisions were made on the basis of factors which related to wider social and political contexts. The failure truly to consider some people with intellectual disabilities as human beings ensures that some of them will continue to be regarded as 'uncontainable' and they will remain in institutions for as long as such places exist.

Note

1 Client Consultation on Relocation. An eight-step process, implemented throughout the closure of Hilltop, by which residents established their preferences for future living arrangements.

References

Bion, W. (1991) *Learning from Experience.* London: Karnac.

Bion, W. (1993) *Second Thoughts: Selected Papers on Psycho-analysis.* London: Karnac.

Day, K. (1994) 'Psychiatric services in mental retardation: Generic or specialized provision.' In N. Bouras (ed.) *Mental Health in Mental Retardation. Recent Advances and Practices.* Cambridge: Cambridge University Press.

Dosen, A. (1994) 'The European view.' In N. Bouras (ed.) *Mental Health in Mental Retardation. Recent Advances and Practices.* Cambridge: Cambridge University Press.

Emerson, E. and Hatton, C. (1996) 'Deinstitutionalisation in the UK and Ireland: Outcomes for service users.' *Journal of Intellectual and Developmental Disabilities 21*, 1, 17–37.

Johnson, K. (1998) *Deinstitutionalising Women. An Ethnographic Study of Institutional Closure.* Melbourne: Cambridge University Press.

Kim, S., Larson, S. and Lakin, K. (2001) 'Behavioural outcomes of deinstitutionalisation for people with intellectual disabilities: A review of US studies conducted between 1980 and 1999.' *Journal of Intellectual and Developmental Disability 26*, 35–50.

Sinason, V. (1992) *Mental Handicap and the Human Condition. New Approaches from the Tavistock.* London: Free Association Books.

Young, L., Sigafoos, J., Suttie, J. and Ashman, A. (1998) 'Deinstitutionalisation of persons with intellectual disabilities: A review of Australian studies.' *Journal of Intellectual and Developmental Disabilities 23*, 2, 155–70.

4

Institutional Death

The Coronial Inquest into the Deaths of Nine Men with Intellectual Disabilities

Ian Freckelton, Australia

In 1996 nine men died in a fire at a large institution in Melbourne, Australia. I was one of the lawyers who was part of a coroner's inquiry to find out what had taken place and why. As part of the inquest I visited the institution where the fire happened. It was a bleak experience on a cold day. I saw the place where the men had lived and died. It was an old building with many doors and passages. There were still many people living in the institution but we only saw them from a distance.

The inquiry found that the fire was started accidentally by a person living in the unit who had got a cigarette lighter. It found that the fire-warning systems were not satisfactory in the unit, that there were delays in contacting the fire brigade and that there were not enough staff on duty to look after the residents' safety. It also found that the staff should have watched the resident who lit the fire more closely because he was known to like lighting fires. As a result of the inquiry, the government spent a lot of money to make institutions safer. But there were many questions that still needed answers after the coroner's inquest. Two of these were: should these men (and other people) have been living in the institution? Would they have been better off in group homes in the community?

On a bleak day in October 1996 a strange procession wended its way through Kew Residential Services ('Kew Cottages'). At the time Kew Cottages accommodated approximately 600 residents with intellectual disabilities, aged between 21 and 68 years, and contained 28 residential units or wards. These were said by those who ran the institution to be designed, as far as possible, to provide a home-like atmosphere. Kew Cottages was originally built in the grounds of Willsmere Hospital in 1887, in Victorian bluestone. It was situated on about 40 hectares of parkland on a picturesque hill overlooking the sprawling expanse of Melbourne (see Lloyd 1987). By 1996 it had experienced a series of changes and expansions, making it one of the larger remaining 'total institutions' in Victoria.

On the day of 'the view', rain threatened, collars were pulled up and minders from Kew Cottages urged everyone to stay together. It was almost as though danger lurked if the visitors did not maintain a strict phalanx. The column was led by the State Coroner and coronial personnel. Others followed: representatives of Kew Cottages and the Department of Human Services, barristers, solicitors, law clerks and, every now and again, a resident who had thwarted the efforts of those who had sought to make the establishment sanitized for the morning. They mostly kept at a respectful distance, sometimes engaging the coroner in slightly stilted conversation. For the most part, the procession and the whole institution were quiet, uncomfortably quiet.

It was a modest walk to Building 37 where, six months before, nine men with intellectual disabilities had perished in a fire that had consumed most of Flat E and damaged parts of Flats B, C and D which made up the building. The unit was a serpentine construction with multiple rooms. It had housed 46 men before the conflagration. The walk was an uncomfortable one, having characteristics in common with a funeral procession but attended too by the realization that it constituted the start of what promised to be one of Victoria's most important coroners' inquests. As the curious cortège progressed deep into the grounds of Kew Cottages, its members looked around expectantly at the institution. We soaked up the mélange of Victorian buildings and post-war prefabricated structures that were home for so many people whom the community never has the opportunity to see. Strange noises that the carers could not quell erupted from some of the buildings as we passed and more than one nose could be observed pressed to the windows. Many of us in the procession wondered what the residents understood about why so many lawyers and officials had descended upon their world. And how much did they know of their colleagues who had died a few months before? Some of the sounds were like howls, some simple shouts. None seemed to be directed particularly toward us. There was a feeling, though, that the whole institution was under constraints, on its best behaviour, until the prying eyes and ears could be ushered off its premises.

When we arrived at Building 37, scene of the fire, a hush fell over the group. This was to be the one opportunity for most of us to acquire a practical perspective on how the building had been constructed, to understand where the men had died, to appreciate where the carers were at the time of the fire, to envisage the scene that must have occurred on the night of 8 April 1996 when flames consumed the building and chaos reigned amongst resident-counts, evacuation procedures and desperate attempts to put out the fire. The quiet was a mark of respect to the deceased, a response to the eeriness of the experience and the start of the legal system formally grinding into action. It initiated a multi-million-dollar inquest that extended over 81 sitting days and did not report until 17 October 1997.

Many memories persist now, years after that visit. For me, counsel for the Office of the Public Advocate of Victoria,[1] the chalked marks of where the men had died and the charred remains of the rooms of Building 37 remain vivid. The men who died, Alan Negri, Joseph Richmond, Adrian Edmunds, Thomas Grant, Shayne Newman, Bruce Haw, Stanley Mathews, Peter Otis and Ronald Aldrige, were hardly ever named during the inquest. This was somewhat symbolic of how their lives had been lived. They were aged between 31 and 61 at the time of their deaths and most had lived at Kew Cottages for many years, some of them for decades. It was possible to see where their beds had been and that a number of the men had crumpled to the floor and, presumably, died of asphyxiation without being able to leave their rooms or escape through the labyrinthine construction to safety. Did they know what was happening? Were they frightened, disorientated? What sounds were there as the smoke became thicker and thicker and the noise of the flames approached? Did they die before the flames engulfed them? What could have been done to avoid such a disaster?

The awfulness of the night some months before was present for each person visiting Kew Cottages on that rainy day, but we all did our best to concentrate upon technical details: the positioning of the bodies, any clues as to where and how the fire might have started, the route of access for the fire officers who had ultimately put the fire out and the functionality of the alarm systems and sprinklers in place on the fateful evening. The vulnerability of the residents was upon all our minds, though, as was the question as to whether it was a breach of trust that had led to the deaths of these men. We looked from the charred remains of the unit toward the nineteenth-century buildings which functioned as the administrative centre for those who ran Kew Cottages, and beyond them to the tall buildings in the city where the Department of Human Services is to be found – the government department with ultimate responsibility for the welfare of people placed in State care because of their intellectual disabilities.

It was clear even then at the view of the death scene that the inquest into the deaths of the nine men at Kew Cottages was going to prove a test for the capacity of the legal system. Could it play a socially constructive role in uncovering how disabled people had died in such dreadful circumstances? What contribution could it make to reducing the likelihood that such a tragedy would be repeated? The coroner's hearing was the only chance for the legal system to play such a role. None of the deceased had dependants, so no civil action was likely or feasible. No identifiable individual had been responsible for starting the fire, save perhaps one of the residents, who was significantly disabled, so no criminal charges were viable. The coroner's inquest was the one opportunity for the relatives of the deceased and the general community to understand how the alarm and sprinkler systems had proved so inadequate, how evacuation procedures could have miscarried, how a fire could have started from what appeared to be a cigarette lighter possessed by one of the residents and how nine men could have perished before the flames were doused. And as the coroner's findings and recommendations themselves do not compel anyone to do anything (Freckelton and Ranson 2005), it was always going be public concern, fanned by media coverage of the inquest, that would decide whether the deaths of the nine men at Kew were going to be the catalyst for change.

Quickly the focus of the inquest shifted toward systemic and mechanistic failures that had made it possible for the fire to start, explained why it had taken so long for the fire alarm to raise a response, why the sprinklers were ineffective and why the intervention of the fire brigade was delayed. The coroner gave leave to the Office of the Public Advocate to participate in the inquest, also to the Kew Cottages and St Nicholas Parents' Association, which purported at least partially to represent the families of the deceased, and to the Villamanta Legal Service, a community legal service which functioned as an advocate for disabled people's rights. In addition, the Departments of Human Services and Infrastructure were both represented by senior counsel in an effort to distance the State of Victoria from any blame. The Metropolitan Fire Brigade also participated in the inquest, maintaining that its members had done all that they could properly do. Builders of the unit, providers of alarm systems, architects, the Health and Community Services Union and individual persons on duty on the night, as well as the resident suspected of having started the fire, were also legally represented.

Each blamed someone else and each maintained that their actions or inactions did not contribute to the causes of the conflagration or the deaths of the deceased. No entity, government department or individual in the course of the inquest assumed any responsibility for the fatalities. Only the State of Victoria (in face of little by way of a forensic alternative) was prepared to admit deficits in the conditions within the unit and that, had proper systems been in place: 'it is likely that the loss of life would have been reduced or prevented' (Johnstone 1997, p.276). Determining whether the deaths were just one of those accidents that can happen (to disabled people who happen to be institutionalized), or whether persons, bodies or institutions culpably contributed to the death, was the task of the coroner.

Many fascinating agendas were played out in the background of the inquest and were sometimes aired in the court. Fundamental to thc Villamanta Legal Service was the issue of whether the men should have been institutionalized at all or whether they should have been looked after in smaller, more normalized houses in the general community. So far as the Public Advocate was concerned, there were major questions too about whether the circumstances of the deceased men's accommodation were suitable in the modern era when people with disabilities should be looked after in as minimally restrictive a way as possible. The Public Advocate argued that there was a direct relationship between the vulnerability of the residents at Kew Cottages, the characteristics of congregate care and the risk of danger to them, realized in the fire. The Parents' Association tended not to question so much whether the men should have been at Kew Cottages, many of the parents having entrusted their children to the care of those running the institution. Rather, the Association maintained that expenditure and monitoring of the residents had been inadequate and a betrayal of their vulnerabilities. Subtexts of whether people with intellectual disabilities should be cared for in traditional institutions such as Kew Cottages formed the backdrop for the focus of the coroner which, by force of statute, had to be upon how the deceased men died, what the causes of the fire and the deaths had been and whether any person or body had contributed to the deaths. For the builders, architects and employees, reputations were on the line. For the government and the institution itself (as well as many other institutions for people with the same and similar disabilities), the spectre loomed of embarrassment, and consequential massive expenditure on accommodation, increased staffing, improved alarm systems and different procedures.

Ultimately, the findings and recommendations of the State Coroner were little less explosive than the fire on the night of 8 April 1996 had been. He found that the nine residents had died from smoke inhalation *and* burns arising from a fire that commenced around 10.49pm on the evening of 8 April 1996 in one of the flats within Unit 30 at Building 37. He found that it was not until 10.56pm that the fire alarm notified the Metropolitan Fire Brigade Communication Centre; the first fire-brigade truck arriving some five minutes later, by which time the fire had broken through to the roof. He determined that the fire had been started by a surviving resident with a cigarette lighter which he had managed to procure on the grounds. The resident had been known to be fascinated by fire and to be a fire-lighting risk. Earlier on the day of the fire, he had been observed by staff to be playing with a lighter which was confiscated but he managed to retain possession of it. Ultimately, it was discovered to be inoperable but the coroner found him to have located another lighter with which he started the fire in bedclothes.

The coroner found that there was no sprinkler system in place within the unit at the time of the fire. It was in the process of being installed but was not operational. Moreover, an effective alarm system was also not in place. It too was going to be installed. Those systems which did exist had a link to the general administrative centre which, in turn, in a cumbersome way, had to communicate back to the unit in order for carers to be alerted that there was a fire on the premises.

The coroner reflected that the State had owed a duty to the staff and to the nine deceased residents, who had not been properly discharged. He found that for ten years the State had been given warning after warning by consultants, experts, personnel and different government bodies as to the inadequacy of the fire-safety system at Kew Cottages. Not only this, but after a strikingly similar fire at the site in 1968 when six psychiatrically ill patients had died, community visitors and the Parents' Association had repeatedly raised concerns about the impoverished state of the safety facilities. Recommended management systems aimed at fire safety had not been adopted; these included re-establishment of the Fire Safety Committee and improvements in fire drills, evacuation procedures and auditing of maintenance.

The coroner found that the response of Kew Cottages had been seriously inadequate and dilatory, meaning that the State of Victoria, through both the

Department of Human Services and through Kew Cottages, had contributed to the fire and the deaths of the nine residents because, despite all the warnings, no proper fire-safety system was in place at the time of the fire. He also found that the State had contributed to the deaths through the Department of Human Services, by its failure to adequately monitor and manage the fire-risk behaviour of the resident who ultimately started the fire. He noted that an increase in staffing levels, especially at night, as had been recommended by consultants, had apparently not been seriously considered – perhaps the expenditure was not thought to be worthwhile from a cost–benefit perspective.

The coroner also found a number of shortcomings, areas deserving of criticism and scope for improvement in the conduct of various consultants and contractors but concluded that they were not so adverse as to justify a finding that they had contributed to the deaths. He commented that:

> Where residents are disabled, elderly or incapacitated, it is essential that the appropriate fire prevention, warning reduction and evacuation procedure is employed... Fire warning and evacuation systems must be developed to cover the needs of the residents, staff and public in the event that a fire develops. Fire reduction and protection systems need to address the ever-present potential for rapid fire conflagration. All of these systems need to consider the disabilities or particular nature of the residents and their environment. In particular, agencies caring for the disabled have a considerable responsibility for their safety. (Johnstone 1997, p.332)

He particularly noted a development that had occurred in the course of the inquest. The State of Victoria, in response to the publicity generated by the coronial hearing, committed $A75.5 million to 'continue the program of fire safety audits and works' in facilities such as Kew Cottages. The coroner commented: 'The extent of the positive work towards improving fire safety along with the implementation of the many recommendations will, no doubt, significantly reduce the chance of such an event recurring' (Johnstone 1997, p.12).

The perspective of hindsight confirms that the inquest was a worthwhile exercise in spite of its length and substantial cost. It provided the impetus for major changes to fire safety for vulnerable persons in many different agencies run and monitored by the State. Governments of both political persuasions were exposed as having been negligent in their care of the residents at Kew Residential Services and many other institutions for those with intellectual disabilities, mental illnesses and age-related vulnerabilities. The incumbent government was embarrassed into spending money on a sector where it and its predecessors had for decades managed successfully to avoid such expenditure. To this extent, the coronial objective of making findings and recommendations directed toward avoiding avoidable deaths was fulfilled.

However, many underlying questions were left unanswered by the inquest. The strength of the process was in its painstaking analysis of mechanistic factors which rendered the residents more vulnerable than they need have been. The weakness of the forum of the coroner's court, with its statutory focus upon causes of death and fire, lay in its failure squarely to deal with the major policy considerations which resulted in the men being housed and cared for in an institutional environment with the characteristics of Kew Cottages. The State Coroner deftly sidestepped many politically and legally sensitive issues, such as those concerning the kinds of residence in which people with disabilities should be housed in the modern era. His shuffle was probably legally correct. The closest he got to these underlying disability issues was to comment that, where locked doors restrict residents, automatic door-latch-release mechanisms should be included in overall layout. No doubt that is so, but the inquest poignantly raised the issue of whether the deceased residents and many other long-time dwellers at Kew Cottages were best housed in such a congregate environment or whether their interests would have been addressed better if the State were persuaded to re-house them in more individualized residences better integrated into the general population. The unit in which the deceased men lived was just one unit in one building in an institution for over 600 people with intellectual disabilities. It continued to function, with some adjustments, on the traditional model of mass care. The fact that the administrative centre for Kew Cottages resided within a nineteenth-century edifice spoke eloquently of the culture.

Such a model of care has traditionally given comfort to family members, to the community and to governments, that those with intellectual disabilities are being looked after, out of harm's way, by professionals knowledgeable about disabilities and accustomed to such responsibilities. But part and parcel of such a model of care is the segregation of people with disabilities in institutionalized environments away from their families and the remainder of the community. Almost inevitably this carries with it the many disadvantages of institutionalization that have been identified for more than half a century. One of these disadvantages is the temptation for those running such establishments, and government departments responsible for monitoring them, to take short cuts with costly outgoings which may not seem to be essential. These can include safety considerations, educational opportunities and individualized measures designed to maximize autonomy, self-realization and potential for enjoyment of life.

Arguably, intrinsic to such congregate care and institutionalized lifestyle is enhanced physical risk. There is a tendency for those responsible for large numbers of people with disabilities who live in the same place to encourage dependency and compliance. It is only through such co-operation and routinized procedures amongst residents that large numbers of persons with vulnerabilities and disabilities can be managed en masse. In Building 37, 46 men lived together. Only two carers were staffing the unit at night. At times there was only one staff member on duty. The design of the unit was convoluted and at times doors were locked to prevent residents wandering around. However, this meant that carers could not be sure of residents' whereabouts. Consequently, those living there, who at any time may have needed to be evacuated in circumstances of emergency, could not be sure whether the doors would be open or whether they would need to wait for a carer to unlock them. It is not known or knowable whether this affected the reactions of the men who were conscious when the smoke began to seep through Building 37 on the night of the fire.

Ironically, the chalked outlines of the huddled bodies of the nine deceased men in Units 30 and 31 have communicated more eloquently to the general community than the men ever had a chance to do during their lives. They raise the issue, years after their death, of whether the men should ever have been living at an institution where their principal identities were congregate rather than individual. Perhaps the question was not one which the Victorian State Coroner was well fitted to answer. But for me, the memory of the noses pressed to the windows as the cortège wended its way through Kew Cottages demands that the question continue to be asked: is there is a better and safer way for people with intellectual disabilities to live than in congregate-care communities, whose era ended some time ago for people with psychiatric illnesses but still persists in many places for those with other disabilities.

Note

1 The Office of the Public Advocate is the body which has statutory responsibility for overseeing the welfare of persons with disabilities in the State of Victoria.

References

Freckelton, I. and Ranson, D. (2005) *Coronial Law and Medicine.* Melbourne: Oxford University Press.

Johnstone, G. (1997) *Inquest Findings, Comments and Recommendations into Fire and Nine Deaths at Kew Residential Services on 8 April 1996.* Melbourne: State Coroner of Victoria.

Lloyd, A. (1987) *Payment by Results: Kew Cottages' First 100 Years 1887–1987.* Melbourne: Kew Cottages and St Nicholas Parents' Association.

5

I've Been in Hospital All My Life

Avis Hunter with Brigit Mirfin-Veitch, New Zealand

I have lived my life in and out of institutions. I've lived in six different institutions and I can't remember all my foster homes. I did not get a choice in where I lived.

I was born in Dunedin, New Zealand on 11 July 1940. My mother named me Avis Maureen Hunter. My mother and father weren't married and my father went to fight in the war before I was born. My mother couldn't afford to look after me. I got sick and ended up in hospital. Then I went to live with a foster family. I was a little baby, just three months old.

I stayed with my foster family until I was four or five years old. They were going to adopt me but the social worker told them not to because I had fits. I was sent to live at an institution where I lived for two years. When I was seven I moved to another institution in a different city. I found it hard to make friends – the other kids were different to me. The staff used to tie me to my bed. I used to cry by myself; people might have hit me if I had cried in front of them. I moved again to another institution in the same city. I liked this one better because I made a friend there. Her name was Connie and she was older than me and she looked after me. I still got scared, though.

When I was 11 I had to go and live with another foster family. I had to work really hard and I did not feel like I was part of the family. I spent a lot of time by myself. Then I lived at an institution called Seacliff. I hated Seacliff. I used to play up a lot and they put me in a straitjacket.

I turned 21 and was moved to another institution, Cherry Farm. I lived there for 27 years before finally getting to live in the community in 1992. Since moving to the community I have found and got to know my family, written a book about my life and met a lot of new friends.

I spent 52 years without a home. My life was spent in and out of institutions. When I wasn't in institutions I lived in foster homes with people who did not want me as part of their family. I was scared a lot in the institution. I have missed out on a lot of things in life but I am not too sad because I have a lot of dreams in life.

Brigit writes: Avis and I were introduced in 1995 when I was asked to help Avis write her life history. At this time, her life-history project was Avis' way of keeping herself occupied while she endured a lengthy and frustrating search for her family. We eventually achieved Avis' goal of documenting the story of her life – a goal that subsequently has motivated her to pursue a host of other literary projects. Avis spent approximately 50 years of her life in a range of institutions in the South Island of New Zealand. When we were asked to write this chapter on Avis' experiences of institutionalization, our first task was to return to her original life history and to begin to expand on her earlier recollections. Our discussions have taken place over endless cups of tea and chocolate biscuits. We have recorded our discussions and then translated them into written narratives. Avis and I continued to develop successive drafts of this chapter until Avis was satisfied that we had achieved an honest account of her experiences of institutionalization. The chapter has been written to reflect Avis' own thoughts and words.

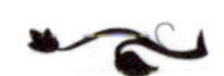

Avis' story

I have always believed that I was found in a basket when I was a little baby and that whoever found me took me to hospital. When I started writing about my life I found out a lot of things I didn't know before. This is because I got to see my records from Child Welfare for the first time and because, finally, I got to meet my family.

My early life

I was born in Dunedin on 11 July 1940. My mother named me Avis Maureen Hunter. My mother's name was Vera and my father's name was George. They were not married. I never got to meet my mother or my father. My father was away fighting in World War Two when I was born. I was only with my mother for a short time, then I became sick and ended up in Dunedin Hospital. I was three months old. My mother was not able to look after me herself, even though she wanted to. I don't know exactly what happened after I ended up in hospital but I do know that I never saw my family again for 56 years.

My first foster home and my first institution

When I was three months old I went to live with my first foster mother. Her name was Elizabeth Smith. I don't remember much about her or her husband because I was too young. She called me Patsy, so for a few years my name was Patsy Smith. We lived in North East Valley. When I was about four or five years old I stopped living with the Smiths. In my records it says I had fits and the social worker told them not to adopt me because of them. I was moved to Nelson. I can't remember the name of the institution that I lived in.

When I was able to look back at my records, I found out my brother Graeme was born at about the time I moved away from the Smiths and went to Nelson. My mother still lived in Dunedin and my father had come back from the war. Graeme and I have the same father. We found a letter in my records that said my mother was still very worried about me but that she was not able to take me back because she did not have a home of her own. She wanted me to be adopted because she felt I would be better off with a family that could afford to take care of me. She thought I was going to be adopted by the Smiths but that never happened. I feel sad about what's happened to me but it's good to know my mother was worried about me.

I spent two years living in Nelson and when I was seven years old I was moved again, this time to Templeton Hospital near Christchurch. I lived in a ward with grown-up women. I didn't like Templeton; I didn't make any friends there. I hated the staff – they used to tie me to my bed.

The other kids were different to me altogether. Some of them couldn't walk or talk. I had to look after myself. I don't know if I cried much. Crying helps some people. I'd run away and cry by myself sometimes. It might have upset people if I'd cried in front of them – they might have hit me.

Growing up

After Templeton I went to live at Sunnyside Hospital; Sunnyside was in Christchurch itself. The best thing about Sunnyside was that I got to meet Connie. Connie was my friend. We were best friends. She was older than me and she looked after me. She had no one to visit and neither did I. Connie used to help me dress and that sort of thing. Connie used to feed the birds in her spare time. We lived in Ward Two. All the women lived in Ward Two.

I used to hide the cat that lived at Sunnyside in my cardigan so I could have a pet to play with. The cat wasn't wild and I really wanted a pet. Connie didn't know I used to do that. Even though I had Connie as a friend I still got scared sometimes. When that happened I would try and climb out of the windows. I do remember Sunnyside as being mostly good now because I had Connie as a friend.

When I was 11 I shifted to a new foster home. My new foster mother's name was Ruby. Ruby was a nurse at Sunnyside when Connie and I lived there. She left work to have a baby. She already had two other children. They were both younger than me. I didn't know the children very well. I didn't know her husband very well either; he wasn't at home very often.

I used to do a lot of work when I was at Ruby's place. I did the gardening, filled the coal buckets, picked fruit and fed the animals. I had to sleep in the sun-porch or wash-house every night. I hardly spoke to Ruby. I was too scared to break windows at her place. I would go to the toilet in the tub in the wash-house because I was too scared to ask her to let me out. She didn't always tell me off but she kept me working very hard. Ruby didn't help me when I had fits, but when I would wake up I would have different clothes on.

I spent a lot of time by myself when I lived at Ruby's. Sometimes Connie would come to stay on weekends. We would talk – Connie was too old to play. She would go back to Sunnyside during the week. Another girl lived there as well. Her name was Miriam. I didn't talk to her much. She did lots of chores around the house as well. Sometimes I would get out and walk along the railway tracks. I would get told off for this. Other times I would go with Ruby and her children to the grandparents' place. I'd wait outside for them.

I stopped living with Ruby because she went away. I went back to Sunnyside. I didn't mind because I liked living at Sunnyside better anyway. I was only at Sunnyside for a little while before I moved back to Dunedin. I was 14. I didn't see Connie again.

After about ten years away from Dunedin I came back. I lived for a short time with a woman called Annie. I can't remember anything about her. I hated being fostered out. It was Welfare. I hate Welfare. I didn't think being fostered out was a good thing and I feel sorry for other children like me.

What happened to me next is quite mixed up. I had to move to the Elliott Street Receiving Home for a short time. Mary Wallace and Mrs Thompson were in charge there. I don't remember much else. It was a yellow building. I used to live in a dorm with four others. The food was all right. I was the oldest one there. I don't know what went on during the day because I went to school. I would come home, have tea and go to bed early.

When I was about 14, I moved from Elliott Street Receiving Home to Seacliff Hospital. I lived at Seacliff after Ward Two had been rebuilt after the Seacliff fire. The ward was painted green. I lived there for seven years. I hated Seacliff.

At Seacliff I was locked up a lot of the time. The staff used to give me paraffin to make me go to the toilet. That was really horrible. I used to wet my bed quite a lot. The staff would help me to change. I would get told off for wetting my bed. I lived in a ward with other women. I didn't make many friends there. I used to play up a lot. I used to break windows and throw things round. I was told to do it. Other patients would say I didn't have the nerve to do things like that. I used to do those things to show them I did have the nerve. I would feel good afterwards. I don't do things like that now because I have grown out of it for good. I didn't know what was right and wrong when I lived there. The staff used to lock me up. Sometimes they would put me in a straitjacket. The nurses in hospitals were often rough with you.

I had a grey-and-black cat that I called Susan when I lived in Seacliff. She would come and hide with me. I don't know what happened to Susan. Sometimes I'd hide under the mattress in the cold weather – wintertime. I'd also hide under the building because I knew that was a really warm place. The hot pipes would keep me warm. When they found me they would get me out.

I would see my visitors in a pink room. I can't remember much about who they were. I've got a photograph of the Seacliff sports day. I didn't like sports. I just watched. The radio was up high. I used to stand up on a chair and listen to 'Aunt Daisy' on it when I was allowed. 'Aunt Daisy' was interesting. When people ran away, the nurses would blow their whistles.

I've been in hospital all my life

When I turned 21 I was no longer under the care of Child Welfare. I think what happened then is that I just moved from Seacliff Hospital to Cherry Farm. I just moved from one hospital to another. Nothing much changed. Just like at the other hospitals I was often scared. I would hide under the building until it was dark. When I came out I would be locked up as punishment. I lived in Cherry Farm for 27 years. Twenty-seven years is a long time and I find it hard to remember much about what I did every day. What I find easier to remember are all the people that I met there and who I think about a lot.

Pearl was a friend of mine. I met her at Cherry Farm – she was a patient there for a while. I remember that her mother and father used to visit her on wet days. Pearl wore a red beret all the time. I used to do the laundry with her. I'd just keep quiet for a start. Then we got to know one another. We used to live together and play cards together at Cherry Farm. She taught me how to play cards. That's why I don't give up playing – because it reminds me.

Jack was another friend of mine – his real name was John. Sometimes I liked him and sometimes I was scared of him. He made me do things that I didn't want to do. He was older than me. Someone dared us to run away together. We had no money but we ran away anyway. We caught the bus outside Cherry Farm; the bus driver let us on even though we had no money. We went to Dunedin. We got off the bus and walked for miles until we found the Leviathan Hotel. We booked a room each. I've always remembered the room number – 132. We stayed the night but the police came and got us in the morning. Jack was locked up and I was taken back to Cherry Farm.

I remember a lot of other people who were important to me when I lived at Cherry Farm. There was Charlie. I used to watch him mow the lawns. Ivan looked after the children – I really liked him. He used to let me out when the nurses locked me up. One person who was very special to me was Reverend Gray. I went to the Presbyterian Church at Cherry Farm; he was the minister there. I used to bang on the church windows until he would let me in. He'd always give me a drink. I would play up a lot when they wouldn't let me see Reverend Gray. I have missed him since I have left Cherry Farm.

One day I heard I was going to move from Cherry Farm. I was happy about that. I was worried that I would not get to see my friends any more, though. I have lost a lot of friends that I knew when I lived in Cherry Farm because I've lost contact with them since I've lived in the community. The good thing that has happened is that I've made a lot of new friends *and* I've finally got to meet my family. I wouldn't want to go back to those hospitals.

Out of the institution

In 1992 I moved out of Cherry Farm. I lived at Wakari Hospital for a while, then I moved into a house in the community. I don't remember much about the move – just that one day I was told that I was shifting. In Cherry Farm I would climb fences. Now I go to Connections on Monday, Wednesday and Friday. I have written and published a book about my life and a book for children. I have also been involved in writing a play based on my life story.

I've got lots of friends now. Some are people from Cherry Farm but most of my friends are people I've met since I have moved out. I like to make new friends and to keep in touch with my old friends. My friends are really important to me.

Finding my family

For my whole life I have lived in foster homes and hospitals, one after the other. Some of the time I have been happy because I have had friends. Other times I have been lonely and scared. All the time I've wanted to know who my people are.

I've always felt lost but I knew that there would be someone in my life. Because I was fostered when I was a very small baby it has been hard to find my family.

On Sunday 4 May 1996 I was given the best news of my life. My family had been found. For a start I didn't think that I would get to meet them. I was just going to write them a letter. Then I found out they were as pleased to find out about me and were coming to meet me the next day.

The first people I met were my brother Graeme and his partner Gail and my two half-sisters Frances and Jocelyn. They told me that I also had another half-sister, Jackie, who lives in the North Island and a half-brother, David, who was killed in an accident before I got to meet him. I also found out that I am an auntie. I didn't expect to have such a big family.

We talked for three hours on our first meeting. I sat and listened to all the things about my family that I had always wanted to know. My brother and sisters brought photos of their families to show me. I showed them the photo that I had of my mother. My brother told me it wasn't my mother. I don't know how long I've had it or who told me it was my mother. I'm glad I found out it wasn't her. I now have another photo of my real mother and I know it is really her.

I knew I had a family somewhere. I feel happier now I've found them. I feel sad about what I've missed out on, though. Both my mother and my father died before I got to meet them and I feel sad about that. I've been crying a lot when I think how close my family was to me and I didn't know them. No one let me know when my mother died because no one knew about me. I don't know if my mother told the rest of the family about me and what had happened to me. I wish I could have met her but she died before I found out who she was.

My sisters used to visit every week and I got to know them really well. Sadly, both my sisters died last year. I was really close to them – they liked me. My brother visits a bit less because he is really busy with work. Sometimes my brother makes me laugh so much I wet my pants. We are really alike. I make sure they have cups of tea whenever they want; I like to be able to give them something when they come.

My life: in and out of institutions

I spent 52 years without a home. My life was spent in and out of institutions. Even when I wasn't living in institutions I wasn't with people who wanted me as part of their family. Some people were nice to me but I never liked living in institutions – I felt trapped. Sometimes I dream about the hospitals I have been in. It can happen any time. When I dream about those places the dreams always wake me up. They are bad dreams. I wake up scared that I am still there. Sometimes they make me laugh and cry at the same time. I see the people I knew when I was there as plain as day.

Water reminds me of Cherry Farm – all the women had to shower together every night. I was scared a lot in the institutions. I would scream a lot. People thought I was being naughty but I was just scared. I would get in the corner and put my hands over my face and no one ever came to comfort me. I'm disappointed that I've never had a job – I never got the chance. Money is not everything in life but I would like to be able to buy clothes. I'm not too sad. I've got all sorts of dreams in life.

6

The Institutions Are Dying, but Are Not Dead Yet

Steven J. Taylor, USA

This chapter looks at something called 'the continuum model of services' for people with intellectual disabilities and at the current disagreements about deinstitutionalization in the USA. The continuum model and a related idea called 'the least restrictive environment' (LRE) became popular in the late 1960s and 1970s. At first, when these ideas were developed, they were forward-looking and led to the development of services outside institutions. But today the continuum and the LRE principle are often used by people who believe we need the institutions and who want segregated services to continue. The chapter looks at the history of the continuum model and LRE principle and points out some of the problems with the ideas behind them. The chapter ends by discussing some of the disagreements about deinstitutionalization today and argues that people need to change the way they think about services and supports for people with intellectual disabilities.

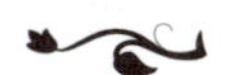

The question of segregation versus integration, or institutions versus the community, was resolved many years ago, in my opinion. I have become much more interested in studying and trying to understand the complexity of life in the community. How can people with intellectual disabilities be supported to participate in the life of the community? How can community services be offered in ways that maximize personal autonomy and choice without jeopardizing health and safety? What kinds of community supports are necessary to enable children with intellectual disabilities to remain with their families? How can we safeguard basic rights without imposing bureaucratic restrictions on community services? What are the characteristics of responsive and effective organizations supporting people with intellectual disabilities and their families?

Although I have long since concluded that institutions have no place in the intellectual disability service system, I am aware that not everyone agrees with this position (see, for example, Erb 1995; Voice of the Retarded 1996, 1997, 2002, 2004). Further, in the USA, deinstitutionalization remains controversial in the media and certain policy circles. Individuals and groups who support institutions defend their position by arguing for the need for a 'continuum' of services (Voice of the Retarded 2004).

In this chapter, I first review the continuum as a concept, building on some of my previous writings on the topic. I then address the continuum of services in the light of current trends and controversies in the field of intellectual disabilities in the USA. In the conclusion I briefly comment on the institution debate and assess the future of the continuum concept.

The continuum as a concept

The concept of the continuum and the associated principle of the 'least restrictive environment' (LRE) have their origins in professional writings and US law (Turnbull and Turnbull 2000; Turnbull *et al.* 1981). US legislative bodies, administrative agencies and courts have relied upon professional literature and testimony in defining the LRE continuum, and professionals have looked to statutes, regulations and court rulings for guidance in providing residential, vocational and educational services for people with intellectual disabilities.

History of the continuum concept

As a conceptual framework for the provision of services, the LRE continuum emerged in the 1960s when leaders in the field began to advocate for the development of a range of special education placements for students with disabilities.

Reynolds (1962) called for a continuum of placements for students with disabilities ranging from the least restrictive to the most restrictive setting. Deno's (1970) 'cascade' of educational placements elaborated on Reynolds' continuum.

In the late 1960s and early 1970s, when US Federal courts began to address the rights of children and adults with disabilities in schools and institutions, they incorporated the notion of an LRE continuum. As Biklen (1982) and Turnbull *et al.* (1981) pointed out, the legal principle of LRE can be traced to constitutional principles such as due process, equal protection and liberty. Biklen (1982) noted that the principle of LRE is deceptively simple: the government must pursue its ends in a manner that least infringes on individual rights. Turnbull *et al.* (1981) described the principle of the least restrictive alternative this way: 'It is a method of limiting government intrusion into people's lives and rights even when the government is acting in an area which is properly open to governmental action' (p.26).

Federal courts in early cases on the right to education and institutional right to treatment ruled that children and adults with disabilities had a right to receive services in the least restrictive environment. In the landmark Wyatt *v.* Stickney (1972) case, Judge Frank Johnson ruled that residents of Alabama's Partlow institution had a constitutional right to the 'least restrictive circumstances necessary to achieve the purposes of habilitation' (p.320). Building on court decisions in the early special education and institutional cases, the US Congress incorporated the LRE continuum into P.L. 94–142, the Education for All Handicapped Children Act of 1975 (now the Individuals with Disabilities Education Act, or IDEA) and the Developmentally Disabled Assistance and Bill of Rights Act of 1975, or DD Act.

With the endorsement of legal bodies, the LRE continuum quickly caught hold in professional circles in the 1970s and 1980s (Blatt *et al.* 1977). By 1976, the Council for Exceptional Children had endorsed the principle that the child with handicaps 'should be educated in the least restrictive environment in which his educational and related needs can be satisfactorily provided' (Bruininks and Lakin 1985, p.16). The American Association on Mental Deficiency, now the American Association on Mental Retardation (AAMR), formed a prestigious task force that issued a definitive analysis of the least restrictive alternative in 1981 (Turnbull *et al.* 1981). Numerous resolutions of TASH, formerly The Association for Persons with Severe Handicaps, have supported LRE, including the 'Resolution on the Redefinition of the Continuum of Services', initially adopted in 1979 and revised in 1986.

Although the idea of the LRE continuum received widespread acceptance in the field, its meaning remained imprecise. The LRE continuum was commonly associated with the most integrated or normalized setting possible, but what was possible could be defined in different ways. Individuals and groups supporting institutionalization have attempted to interpret this concept to justify the continued segregation of people with intellectual disabilities: 'an individual's needs may mean that his/her least restrictive environment is a developmental center'[1] (Voice of the Retarded 1997).

The residential continuum

Since its earliest conceptualization, the LRE continuum has been defined operationally in terms of an ordered sequence of placements that vary according to the degree of restrictiveness. Turnbull *et al.* (1981) described the least restrictive alternative as a hierarchical rank ordering of alternatives:

> the government (or person, family, or professional) presumes that there is a generally accepted hierarchy of placements, treatments, or interventions and that any given one is clearly rank ordered as more or less restrictive. (p.17)

A common way of representing the continuum was a straight line running from the least to the most restrictive environment or a hierarchical cascade of placement options (Hitzing 1980; Reynolds 1962; Schalock 1983). The most restrictive placements were also the most segregated and offered the most intensive services; the least restrictive placements were the most integrated and independent and offered the least intensive services. The assumption was that every person with an intellectual disability could be located somewhere along this continuum based on individual needs. If and when the person developed additional skills, he or she could transition to a less restrictive placement (Hitzing 1987). Figure 6.1 depicts a traditional continuum model of residential services.

The residential continuum ran from public institutions, as the most restrictive environment, to independent living, as the least restrictive environment. In most discussions, an 'institution' has been defined as a large (16 or more residents) State residential facility in which people with intellectual disabilities were cut off or segregated from society. Common names for public institutions have included 'State hospital', 'training school' and 'developmental centre'. 'Community' has generally been understood to mean a facility or home located in ordinary housing or a residential neighbourhood. Between these extremes were nursing homes and private institutions, community Intermediate Care Facilities for the Mentally

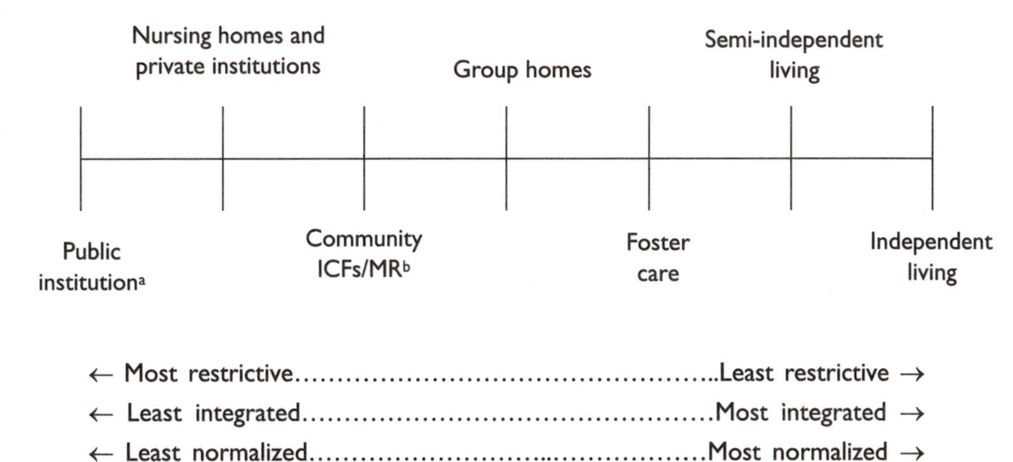

Figure 6.1: The traditional residential continuum

Retarded (ICFs/MR; in the US a Federal-State funding programme), group homes, foster care and semi-independent living.

The residential continuum was based on the assumption that people with intellectual disabilities would move progressively to less and less restrictive settings and ideally to independent living. For those who supported institutionalization, institutions would prepare people with intellectual disabilities to move to less restrictive settings in the community (Aines and Knapp 1986; Crissey and Rosen 1986; Walsh and McCallion 1987). Walsh and McCallion (1987) wrote:

> Restructuring institutions demands a shift in emphasis from relentless custody to transitional programming. Proactive, habilitative training must

---

a In the USA, public institutions are commonly defined as large (16 or more residents) State-operated public facilities. Public institutions share the characteristics of 'total institutions' as described by Goffman (1961): 'A total institution may be defined as a place of residence and work where a large number of like-situated individuals, cut off from the wider society for an appreciable period of time, together lead an enclosed, formally administered round of life' (p.xiii). Of course, private institutions and smaller 'community-based' facilities can also fit Goffman's definition of a total institution.

b The ICF/MR (Intermediate Care Facilities for the Mentally Retarded) programme is a joint Federal and State programme that funds facilities providing medical or rehabilitative services to people with developmental disabilities. The ICF/MR programme funds both institutions and 'small' (typically 6–15 persons) community facilities. Community ICFs/MR are generally more highly regulated and medically oriented than other community settings.

> be unstintingly directed toward imparting skills needed by clients to move continuously to less restrictive settings, beginning with the most basic skills in the institution and ending in successful, continued community placement. (pp.233–4)

In the 1980s, an increasing number of researchers and professionals began to argue for a redefinition of the traditional continuum (Bronston 1980; Galloway 1980; Haring and Hansen 1981; Hitzing 1980, 1987; Lakin *et al.* 1986; Schalock 1983). According to the new vision, the traditional continuum would be replaced by a range of least restrictive settings in the community.

Conceptual flaws in the continuum

As a conceptual framework for the design of services for people with intellectual disabilities, the LRE continuum is seriously flawed. For people with severe disabilities, in particular, this concept is full of pitfalls. Five of the most serious flaws in the LRE continuum are reviewed here (also see Taylor 1988).

The LRE continuum confuses segregation, on the one hand, with intensity of services, on the other. As indicated in Figure 6.1, the continuum concept equates segregation with the most intensive services and integration with the least intensive services. Implicit in the concept is the assumption that the least restrictive, most integrated settings will not provide the intensive services needed by people with severe disabilities.

When viewed from this perspective, it follows that people with severe disabilities will require the most restrictive and segregated settings. Herein lies the flaw: segregation and integration, on the one hand, and intensity of services, on the other, are separate dimensions. Any health-related, educational or habilitative service that can theoretically be provided in a segregated setting can be provided in a integrated setting.

Historically, of course, the most segregated settings provided the least intensive services (Blatt and Kaplan 1966; Blatt, Ozolins and McNally 1979; Taylor and Blatt 1999). When Blatt and Kaplan (1966, p.5) published their photographic exposé of institutions in the 1960s, average expenditures at institutions in the US stood at $4.55 per person per day; medical and educational services were few and far between. Today, over 30 years later, the situation has changed. Institutions capture a disproportionate share of expenditures on services for people with intellectual disabilities. In 2002, average per resident daily expenditures in large public residential facilities in the US had soared to $344.51 (Prouty,

Smith and Lakin 2003). In order to attempt to comply with Federal requirements, US institutions have hired scores of health-care workers, therapists and professionals.

The debate over institutions versus the community is not a debate over whether some people require intensive services and supports. The debate is whether certain people must forfeit their place in the community as a condition of receiving services. The continuum concept obscures the nature of the issues at hand.

The LRE continuum sanctions infringements on basic human rights. LRE is a seductive concept; government should act in a manner that least restricts the rights and liberties of individuals. When applied categorically to people with intellectual disabilities, the LRE principle sanctions infringements on basic rights to freedom and community participation. The question implied by the LRE continuum is not *whether* the rights of people with intellectual disabilities should be restricted, but *to what extent.*

The principle of LRE may be appropriate in the case of criminal or commitment proceedings in which some level of restriction may arguably be justified (Turnbull and Turnbull 1978; Turnbull *et al.* 1981). People with or without disabilities who have been proven to have committed crimes through proceedings well established in the US judicial system or English Common Law should expect to have their rights restricted. Linked to the provision of services to people with intellectual disabilities, a principle that sanctions the restriction of rights cannot be justified. It is not a crime to have an intellectual disability, and no one should be denied the opportunity to live and participate in community life on this basis – even if parents, guardians or loved ones desire this. In regard to providing services, as distinguished from exercising social control, people with intellectual disabilities should be able to live, work and go to school in the same settings as other people.

The LRE continuum is based on a 'readiness model'. Inherent in the continuum concept is the requirement that people with intellectual disabilities must earn the right to move to the least restrictive, most integrated settings. The person must 'get ready' or 'be prepared' to live in the community, with residential programmes designed as 'transitional'. As Hitzing (1980) noted in an early critique of the continuum concept:

> The notion was that a person moved into the residential system initially by being placed in a nursing home or large group home. Once clients 'shaped

> up,' they 'graduated' to a smaller group home. If they learned certain skills in the group home, they 'graduated' to a more independent placement unit. (p.84)

Institutions do not and cannot prepare people to live in the community. Living in an institution – the rhythms and routines of life, behavioural expectations, the nature of role models – is fundamentally different from ordinary community life.

Even if people moved smoothly through the continuum, their lives would be a series of stops between transitional placements. This would destroy any sense of home and disrupt relationships with roommates, neighbours and friends.

The LRE continuum directs attention to physical settings rather than to the services and supports people need to live successfully in the community. As Gunnar Dybwad (personal communication, February 1985) once stated: 'Every time we identify a need in this field, we build a building.' The LRE continuum emphasizes facilities and physical environments. Services are confused with bricks and mortar. As a consequence, 'independent living' – the 'least restrictive' step in the continuum – has often been associated with minimal services, even neglect. Instead of focusing on buildings and facilities, we should be working to make sure that supports are sufficient to enable people with intellectual disabilities to live in ordinary homes, neighbourhoods and communities.

The continuum's emphasis on physical environments is reflected in the field's preoccupation with the size of residential facilities (Landesman-Dwyer 1981; for a discussion of the field's obsession with trying to determine the optimal size of facilities, see Rothman and Rothman 1984). It seems self-evident that smaller settings will provide more personalized care and are less susceptible to the 'block treatment' associated with institutions (King, Raynes and Tizard 1971). Research in Australia (Stancliffe 1997), Norway (Tøssebro 1995) and North America (Stancliffe and Abery 1997) has demonstrated that small living units (one to five persons) have a significant impact on self-determination and opportunities for privacy. Yet a focus on size detracts attention from the need to support people with intellectual disabilities to live in ordinary homes as opposed to 'home-like' facilities.

The concept of the continuum emerged in an era in which people with intellectual disabilities and their families were offered segregation or nothing at all. The early proponents of the concept were extremely forward-looking for their time. For example, Reynolds (1962), who presented one of the earliest and clearest formulations of the concept, also helped to popularize the notion of 'mainstreaming' students with disabilities in public schools. The continuum was used to create opportunities for integration when few existed. It is ironic, therefore, that the continuum concept is used today to support institutionalization.

The continuum as controversy

As a conceptual framework for the design of intellectual disability services, the LRE continuum has fallen upon difficult times. Whereas the 'least restrictive environment' and the 'continuum' once appeared routinely in the titles of State planning documents (State of New York Office of Mental Retardation and Developmental Disabilities 1987), professional journal articles (Biklen 1982; Peck and Semmel 1982) and leading texts and monographs in the field (Bruininks and Lakin 1985; Turnbull *et al.* 1981), it has become increasingly difficult to find references to these concepts in the research or policy literature. The field of intellectual disabilities is dominated today by a new set of concepts and ideas: self-determination (Nerney, Crowley and Kappel 1997) and individual budgeting (Moseley, Gettings and Cooper 2003), person-centred planning (O'Brien and Mount 2003), support paradigms (Coulter 1996; Luckasson *et al.* 2002; Smull and Bellamy 1991), quality of life (Goode 1994; Schalock 1996a, 1996b; Schalock and Alonso 2002) and others.

Yet, the continuum – as a word and conceptual framework – is not dead yet. It has become, in certain circles, a synonym for public institutions for people with intellectual disabilities. Thus, a concept that was developed to expand community options for people with intellectual disabilities has been appropriated by those who would seek to justify the continued existence of State-operated 'developmental centres' and 'training schools'. The late Burton Blatt predicted as much in 1979 (Blatt *et al.* 1979, p.4) when he commented on the 'camouflage of benign vocabulary' used to defend institutions.

So now we find ourselves in the early stages of the new millennium. What is the status of the institution-versus-community debate? Before I attempt to answer this question, I want to clarify the nature of the discussion: as a matter of public policy, should we, as a society – whether the US, Canada, Australia, New Zealand, Great Britain, Iceland, Sweden or elsewhere – put our resources into supporting people with intellectual disabilities to live in the community or should we permit our resources to be used to support institutionalization? The debate is *not* about whether any group has the right to isolate themselves from other people. For various reasons, certain groups of people – based on religious persuasion, ethnic background or sexual orientation – choose to cut off relations with the broader society. As long as people do so freely and voluntarily, this is their right. The debate *is* about whether public policy and resources should support people with intellectual disabilities to live among us or to be put away, at the discretion of family members or guardians.

The emerging consensus

The earliest critics of institutions in the 1960s (Blatt and Kaplan 1966; Dybwad 1964) were advocates of institutional reform with an expansion of services in the community. By the 1970s, a small but growing number of leaders in the field had concluded that institutional reform was hopeless. As Blatt (Blatt *et al.* 1979) wrote:

> If there is hope in what we have learned in our examination of institutionalization, it is not in any improvement of institutional life – imprisonment and segregation can be made more comfortable, but they can never be made into freedom and participation. (p.5)

Today, most major organizations and leaders in intellectual disabilities support community living. As of 2004, 183 organizations had endorsed the Center on Human Policy's *The Community Imperative* declaration, a statement supporting the right of all people with disabilities to community living.

National trends in residential services parallel this prevailing opinion. From 1967 to 2002, the populations of US public institutions declined from 194,650 (Prouty and Lakin 1997) to 44,343 (Prouty *et al.* 2003). Just as striking as the decline in institutional populations in the US has been the pace of institutional closures. From 1960 to 2002, states closed 168 institutions for people with intellectual disabilities. Nine states and the District of Columbia no longer operate any institutions.

Both prevailing opinion and national trends are on the side of community inclusion. This does not mean that all controversies over institutions, or the 'continuum', have disappeared.

The future of the controversy

Controversy over the role of institutions will probably continue in the near future. Every now and then institutional proponents will find a receptive audience among media representatives, elected officials or other groups in their efforts to discredit community living.

Yet this controversy will not continue indefinitely. People with disabilities are increasingly visible in communities throughout North America and accepted as equal members. Attitudes toward people with disabilities are slowly but surely changing (Taylor and Bogdan 1993). The Americans with Disabilities Act is but one example of increased recognition that people with disabilities should have the right to participate fully in community life. Attempts to exclude people with intellectual disabilities from this broader trend will not be successful.

Even more immediate, the institutions are gradually losing their constituencies. The growing number of states that have closed their institutions no longer have active institutional proponents. In other states, the populations of institutions are ageing. From 1977 to 2002, the percentage of institutionalized persons age 40 or older in the US grew from 22.9 per cent to 64.6 per cent (Prouty *et al.* 2003). Most striking is the dramatic decline in the number of children living at public institutions. From 1977 to 2002, the number of children and youths in US institutions decreased from over 54,000 to approximately 1478 (Prouty *et al.* 2003).

In contrast to past generations, families today have benefited from a public education for their children with intellectual disabilities and increasing availability of family-support services. Few families who have supported their children to participate in the community will be willing to have their sons and daughters placed in institutions when they reach adulthood. If deinstitutionalization is controversial among families, it is not because any significant number want their sons and daughters placed in institutions; it is because some do not want their children placed out of such places.

The institutions are dying. This is what has sparked current controversies over institutionalization or the continuum. As the institutions continue to die, however, so will the controversies.

Discussion

For those of us committed to the community, and who have worked to strengthen the quality and responsiveness of community services and family supports, the institution-versus-community debate is a distraction. An earlier generation of leaders such as Gunnar Dybwad, Burton Blatt and Wolf Wolfensberger spent a good part of their careers unmasking the nature of institutions. It is long past time to move on to other issues and challenges. However, if need be, community advocates will come forward to re-argue the issue and will be prepared to marshal the same kinds of arguments and evidence to support the community position. Unfortunately, this will come at the expense of efforts to expose and rectify bad policy decisions made in the name of the 'community'.

What is the future of the LRE continuum? Because it has come to be associated with a pro-institution position, the continuum, as a word, is falling into disrepute. Yet the LRE continuum continues to serve as a conceptual foundation for the design of services for people with intellectual disabilities. Whether explicit or implicit, the assumption is that there should be a range of service options or placements that vary in integration and opportunities for independence – or restrictiveness, self-determination and so on – and that severity of disability should be the determining factor in deciding a person's living situation. As long as this assumption is unchallenged, approaches such as supported living, home ownership, self-directed supports and individualized funding will simply represent new slots on the least restrictive end of the continuum. What is needed are not new slots but changes in how services and supports are conceptualized.

Acknowledgements

The preparation of this chapter was supported in part through subcontract from the Research and Training Center on Community Living at the University of Minnesota awarded to the Center on Human Policy. The Research and Training Center on Community Living is funded by the US Department of Education, Office of Special Education and Rehabilitative Services, National Institute on Disability and Rehabilitation Research (NIDRR). Members of the Center are encouraged to express their opinions; however, these do not necessarily represent the official position of NIDRR and no endorsement should be inferred. This chapter is a significantly shortened and revised version of an article originally published in the *Journal of Intellectual and Developmental Disability* (Taylor 2001). Permission to use this material was granted by the editor Dr Roger J. Stancliffe.

Note

1 In the US, insitutions are often referred to as 'developmental centres'.

References

Aines, J.P. and Knapp, C.W. (1986) 'Institutions as community resources for vocational habilitation.' In M.S. Crissey and M. Rosen (eds) *Institutions for the Mentally Retarded.* Austin, TX: Pro-Ed.

Biklen, D. (1982) 'The least restrictive environment: Its application to education.' In G. Melton (ed.) *Child and Youth Services.* New York: Haworth.

Blatt, B., Bogdan, R., Biklen, D. and Taylor, S.J. (1977) 'From institution to community: A conversion model.' In E. Sontag (ed.) *Educational Programming for the Severely and Profoundly Handicapped.* Reston, VA: Council for Exceptional Children.

Blatt, B. and Kaplan, F. (1966) *Christmas in Purgatory: A Photographic Essay on Mental Retardation.* Boston: Allyn & Bacon.

Blatt, B., Ozolins, A. and McNally, J. (1979) *The Family Papers.* New York: Longman.

Bronston, W. (1980) 'Matters of design.' In T. Appolloni, J. Cappuccilli and T.P. Cooke (eds) *Towards Excellence: Achievements in Residential Services for Persons with Disabilities.* Baltimore, MD: University Park Press.

Bruininks, R.H. and Lakin, K.C. (eds) (1985) *Living and Learning in the Least Restrictive Environment.* Baltimore, MD: Paul H. Brookes.

Coulter, D. (1996) 'Prevention as a form of support: Implications for the new definition.' *Mental Retardation 34,* 2, 108–116.

Crissey, M.S. and Rosen, M. (eds) (1986) *Institutions for the Mentally Retarded.* Austin, TX: Pro-Ed.

Deno, E. (1970) 'Special education as developmental capital.' *Exceptional Children 37,* 229–37.

Dybwad, G. (1964) *Challenges in Mental Retardation.* New York: Columbia University Press.

Erb, R.G. (1995) 'Where, oh where, has common sense gone? (Or if the shoe doesn't fit, why wear it?)' *Mental Retardation 33,* 3, 197–8.

Galloway, C. (1980) 'The "continuum" and the need for caution.' Unpublished manuscript.

Goffman, E. (1961) *Asylums: Essays on the Social Situation of Mental Patients and Other Inmates.* London: Peregrine Books.

Goode, D. (1994) *Quality of Life for Persons with Disabilities: International Perspectives and Issues.* Cambridge, MA: Brookline Books.

Haring, N.G. and Hansen, C.L. (1981) 'Perspectives in communitization.' In C.L. Hansen (ed.) *Severely Handicapped Persons in the Community.* Seattle, WA: Program Development Assistance System.

Hitzing, W. (1980) 'ENCOR and beyond.' In T. Appolloni, J., Cappuccilli and T.P. Cooke (eds) *Towards Excellence: Achievements in Residential Services for Persons with Disabilities.* Baltimore, MD: University Park Press.

Hitzing, W. (1987) 'Community living alternatives for persons with autism and severe behavior problems.' In D.J. Cohen and A. Donnellan (eds) *Handbook of Autism and Pervasive Developmental Disorders.* New York: John Wiley.

King, R., Raynes, N. and Tizard, J. (1971) *Patterns of Residential Care: Sociological Studies in Institutions for Handicapped Children.* London: Routledge & Kegan Paul.

Lakin, K.C., Hill, B.K., Bruininks, R.H. and White C.C. (1986) 'Residential options and future implications.' In W.E. Kiernan and J.A. Stark (eds) *Pathways to Employment for Adults with Developmental Disabilities.* Baltimore, MD: Paul H. Brookes.

Landesman-Dwyer, S. (1981) 'Living in the community.' *American Journal of Mental Deficiency 86,* 3, 223–34.

Luckasson, R., Borthwick-Duffy, S., Buntix, W.H.E., Coulter, D.L., Craig, E.M., Reeve, A., Schalock, R.L., Snell, M.E., Spitalnik, D., Spreat, S. and Tasse, M.J. (2002) *Mental Retardation: Definition, Classification, and Systems of Support* (10th edition). Washington, DC: American Association on Mental Retardation.

Moseley, C.E., Gettings, R.M. and Cooper, R. (2003) *Having it Your Way: Understanding State Individual Budgeting Strategies.* Alexandria, VA: National Association of State Directors of Developmental Disabilities Services, Inc.

Nerney, T., Crowley, R.F. and Kappel, B. (1997) *An Affirmation of Community, a Revolution of Vision and Goals: Creating a Community to Support all People Including those with Disabilities.* Keene, NH: Monadnock Developmental Services.

O'Brien, J. and Mount, B. (2003) *Person-centered Direct Support.* Toronto: Inclusion Press.

Peck, C.A. and Semmel, M.I. (1982) 'Identifying the least restrictive environment (LRE) for children with severe handicaps: Toward an empirical analysis.' *The Journal of The Association for Persons with Severe Handicap 7,* 1, 56–63.

Prouty, R.W. and Lakin, K.C. (eds) (1997) *Residential Services for Persons with Developmental Disabilities: Status and Trends through 1996.* Minneapolis: University of Minnesota, Research and Training Center on Community Living, Institute on Community Integration.

Prouty, R.W., Smith, G. and Lakin, K.C. (eds) (2003) *Residential Services for Persons with Developmental Disabilities: Status and Trends through 2002.* Minneapolis: University of Minnesota, Research and Training Center on Community Living, Institute on Community Integration.

Reynolds, M. (1962) 'A framework for considering some issues in special education.' *Exceptional Children 28,* 367–70.

Rothman, D.J. and Rothman, S.M. (1984) *The Willowbrook Wars.* New York: Harper & Row.

Schalock, R.L. (1983) *Services for Developmentally Disabled Adults.* Baltimore, MD: University Park Press.

Schalock, R.L. (ed.) (1996a) *Quality of Life Volume I: Conceptualization and Measurement.* Washington, DC: American Association on Mental Retardation.

Schalock, R.L. (ed.) (1996b) *Quality of Life Volume II: Application to Persons with Disabilities.* Washington, DC: American Association on Mental Retardation.

Schalock, R. and Alonso, M.A.V. (2002) *Handbook on Quality of Life for Human Service Practitioners.* Washington, DC: American Association on Mental Retardation.

Smull, M.W. and Bellamy, T.G. (1991) 'Community services for adults with disabilities: Policy challenges in the emerging support paradigm.' In L.H. Meyer, C.A. Peck and L. Brown (eds) *Critical Issues in the Lives of People with Severe Disabilities.* Baltimore, MD: Paul H. Brookes.

Stancliffe, R.J. (1997) 'Community living-unit size, staff presence, and residents' choice making.' *Mental Retardation 35,* 1, 1–9.

Stancliffe, R.J. and Abery, B.H. (1997) 'Longitudinal study of deinstitutionalization and the exercise of choice.' *Mental Retardation 35,* 3, 159–69.

State of New York Office of Mental Retardation and Developmental Disabilities (1987) *Strengthening the Continuum 1987–1990.* Albany, NY: Author.

Taylor, S.J. (1988) 'Caught in the continuum: A critical analysis of the principle of the least restrictive environment.' *Journal of the Association for Persons with Severe Handicaps 13,* 1, 45–53.

Taylor, S.J. (2001) 'The continuum and current controversies in the USA.' *Journal of Intellectual and Developmental Disability 26,* 1, 15–33.

Taylor, S.J. and Blatt, S.D. (1999) *In Search of the Promised Land: The Collected Papers of Burton Blatt.* Washington, DC: American Association on Mental Retardation.

Taylor, S.J. and Bogdan, R. (1993) 'Promises made and promises to be broken.' In P. Wehman (ed.) *The ADA Mandate for Social Change.* Baltimore, MD: Paul H. Brookes.

Tøssebro, J. (1995) 'Impact of size revisited: Relation of number of residents to self-determination and deprivatization.' *American Journal on Mental Retardation 100*, 1, 59–67.

Turnbull, H.R. and Turnbull, A.P. (1978) *Free Appropriate Public Education: Law and Implementation.* Denver, CO: Love.

Turnbull, H.R. and Turnbull, A.P. (2000) *Free Appropriate Public Education: The Law and Children with Disabilities* (6th edition). Denver, CO: Love Publishing Company.

Turnbull, R., with Ellis, J.W., Boggs, E.M., Brookes, P.O. and Biklen D.P. (eds) (1981) *Least Restrictive Alternatives: Principles and Practices.* Washington, DC: American Association on Mental Deficiency.

Voice of the Retarded (1996) *Center of Excellence Concept.* http://www.world2u.com/~pmay/vor9.html

Voice of the Retarded (1997) *VOR Position on 'De-institutionalization.'* http://www.world2u.com/~pmay/vor11.html

Voice of the Retarded (2002) *Executive Summary: Institutional and Community-based Systems for People with Mental Retardation: A Review of the Cost Literature.* http://www.vor.net/

Voice of the Retarded (2004) *Speaking Out for Choices.* http://www.vor.net/about.html

Walsh, K.K. and McCallion, P. (1987) 'The role of the small institution in the community services continuum.' In R.F. Antonak and J.A. Mulick (eds) *Transitions in Mental Retardation, Volume 3: The Community Imperative Revisited.* Norwood, NJ: Ablex.

Wyatt *v.* Stickney, 344 F. Supp. 387, 390 (M.D. Ala., N.D.) (1972).

PART II

Moving Out

7

It's Never Too Late

Thomas F. Allen with Rannveig Traustadóttir
and Lisa Spina, USA

When I was 70 years old I decided I wanted to move out of the institution. I wanted to move into a group home in the community. My friends encouraged me but my brother Neal did not like the idea. He thought I was too old and frail to move. This was difficult for me because Neal had always helped me and I could not move out of the institution without his consent. It was a great disappointment. I wanted my freedom.

A short time later I joined a group of people at the institution who were preparing a lawsuit to force the state to release us from the institution and allow us to live in the community. The lawyer helped me get in touch with the director of residential community services and they accepted my application for a place in one of their group homes. But there was no space available so I had to wait.

With the lawyer's help I made a statement to take to court. The judge ruled that I should be released from the institution. I was very happy and wanted to move right away. But I had no place to go so I had to stay another year and a half while I waited for a place in the community.

In 1985 I was offered a place in an apartment in downtown Syracuse. I went for a visit overnight and liked it very much. I had visited other group homes and did not like any of them. This was the best place I had been to and I decided to look no further. I packed my few belongings and moved. It had taken two and a half years of hard work to get out of the institution. Finally it was happening.

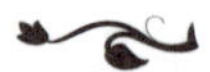

Tom Allen's story is continued from Chapter 1. Please see pp.34–35and the Epilogue to Thomas F. Allen's Life Story on p.274 for a description of how the story was told and written.

Tom's story *continued*

It was 1982. I was 70 years old and had spent almost 60 years in institutions when I decided to move out. I wanted to see if I could move into a group home in the community. I began talking about this with my friends and they encouraged me to do something about it. I also talked to Neal but he did not like the idea. He thought I was too old and felt my health was too fragile. Neal believed I needed to be in the institution. This was very difficult for me. Neal had always supported me and helped me with my moves but now he refused and I could not be released from Syracuse Developmental Center (SDC) without his consent. I was very disappointed and became depressed for a while. I wanted to be free. Free to participate in the life outside. Free from the violence in the institution. Free to do the things I wanted to do. Free to make my dream come true. I wanted my freedom. I did not want to be locked up any longer.

The lawsuit

A short while later a lawyer came to a resident government meeting. She talked about a court case that some of the people at SDC wanted to join. It was a Federal suit to force the state to release us from SDC and allow us to live in the community. This was my chance. I talked to her and she was interested in my case. I decided to join the suit. It was a very difficult decision for me. Neal did not want me to move out of SDC and I had never gone against him before. I was afraid of what he would do or say. But all he said was that if I really wanted this then I should do it, although he still believed it would be better for me to stay in SDC. I was relieved to hear his reaction.

The lawyer helped me get in contact with the director of United Cerebral Palsy for Residential Community Services. The director came to SDC to talk to me and I filled out an application. I got a letter saying I was eligible for placement in their programme. They had no openings in their apartments at the time but they said they would contact me when anything became available. I was disappointed but I could not do anything but wait.

The lawyer wanted me to make a statement to take to a judge. Two friends of mine, who had been working in Craig Developmental Center when I was there and were now working at SDC, took me to her office. The lawyer asked me a lot of questions and then she prepared the following statement (which she called an affidavit) based on what I told her:

> I was first institutionalized at Rome Developmental Center in 1914 and returned to my parents' home in 1919, where I remained until about 1927. In 1927, I was re-institutionalized at Rome until 1973.
>
> While I was at Craig Developmental Center and Rome Developmental Center, I was subjected to assaults at the hands of residents and staff. I was left unattended in a manual wheelchair for hours; I was placed on the floor in a bathroom and left alone all day without meals; I was left in a large room that reeked of urine and feces for entire days with other residents.
>
> None of us had programming or activities to occupy our time and our minds. The majority of the other residents were mentally retarded, and I could not even communicate with them.
>
> Many of the residents were not clothed. I had to rely on other residents to dress me. All this time, I was not provided with education or training. I taught myself by using 'talking tapes.' I taught myself daily living skills such as eating and dressing. I have never had privacy except when my friends have taken me out of the institution. I never even had personal belongings until I was 48 years old.
>
> I have been assaulted by other residents and neglected by staff of the Syracuse Developmental Center on numerous occasions.
>
> My glasses have been broken by other residents three or four times. My money and clothing have been stolen from me repeatedly. During mealtimes, food has been taken from me and/or thrown at me.
>
> During November 1982, I was attacked by a resident and suffered an eye injury. During January 1983, a resident hit me in the face three or four times and I slid out of my wheelchair onto the floor and could not get up. I remained on the floor for 15 or 20 minutes before a staff person came to help me.

I have been left on the toilet without assistance from staff on several occasions, which resulted in me being late for work. My electric wheelchair is broken more often than not, and, as a consequence, I am dependent upon others for my mobility.

I spend a great deal of time in my room because I am afraid of physical attacks by other residents against whom SDC staff provide me no protection.

I am a very religious man. I have always wanted to attend church services and receive baptism, but was not given the opportunity to do so until my friends, Walt and Linda Priest, arranged for my baptism in 1981.

I have been frequently disappointed by the state's broken promise to find a home in the community for me. This has been the worst indignity and disappointment I have suffered.

I live in constant fear of assault at SDC. My health is failing. I am often depressed; I worry about whether I will ever live in the community before I die. I have had trouble sleeping at night. I have to hide in my room to get away from other residents who have assaulted me. I feel that I deserve some dignity and a normal life in my last years on this earth and I am afraid I may die in an institution.

I urge the court to grant my motion for a preliminary injunction and allow me the opportunity to live my last years in dignity, in the community.

In court

We took my statement to Federal court in Syracuse. I saw the judge in his chambers. He seemed to be interested in my case and we talked about 15 or 20 minutes. He said he would take the case and scheduled a court date. The morning I went to court I was all dressed up and was accompanied by my lawyer and my two friends. My case was the first to be heard. The SDC people were there also. They discussed my case for about two hours. The judge listened to both sides. He asked a lot of questions but he only asked me a few. He wanted to know why I wanted to leave SDC. I told the judge I wanted to better myself and I thought it would be better for me to live in the community. I wanted to be able to go places and do things that I wanted to do. At SDC I could not do much of what I wanted and I often had to go places I did not want to go. I was a 71-year-old man who wanted to make my own decisions. I had never been allowed to do that.

The judge ruled that I should be released from SDC. I was very happy and wanted to move out of SDC right away. But I had no place to move to. I had to stay about a year and a half while I waited for a place in the community.

Moving out

Finally in February of 1985 I got a letter from United Cerebral Palsy. They had good news! They had an opening at an apartment on South Clinton Street downtown Syracuse. I was told I could come and try it out overnight to see if I liked it.

In all my years at institutions I knew what to expect but this change was something very different to what I had experienced before. The apartment was in downtown Syracuse, on the sixteenth floor of the Clinton Plaza Apartments. One afternoon in early March 1985 I went there for a visit with a staff person from SDC who was my advocate and my friend. I was going to stay overnight to check things out. I met the three other people who lived there: two women and one man. The apartment impressed me. It seemed more like a home than SDC or any of the other places I had been. The manager of the apartment showed me and my advocate around. There were two bedrooms, two bathrooms, a living room, a dining room, a kitchen and an office for the staff. The furniture looked cosy and comfortable, and I was already beginning to think it looked like home to me. 'A home at last!' I thought to myself.

I don't remember what we had for dinner that night but I remember having a warm feeling. I almost felt like I was a part of a family because I was not used to eating with so few people. After dinner we all watched TV until about ten o'clock. One of the resident counsellors, which is what the staff at the apartment are called, helped me get ready for bed and it was a good feeling to say good night to my roommate, knowing I was not at SDC that night. I felt very unsafe at SDC and didn't sleep well there.

My roommate was a peaceful, gentle man, a little younger than I. He had a good sense of humour and I really liked him. We hit it off from the start. His disability was similar to mine. He used a wheelchair and had difficulties speaking but we could understand each other.

The next morning I was given a shower and dressed. I ate breakfast with some of the residents and staff members. It was nice sitting at a table with three or four other people in a family setting. By ten o'clock, when someone from SDC came to take me back, I had made up my mind: I wanted to move into the apartment at Clinton Street. I had been to visit a few group homes and none of them had looked good to me. This was the best place I had been to and I decided to look no further.

It didn't take me long to pack what few belongings I had: my clothes, my rocking chair and my family pictures. It took two and a half years of hard work to get out of SDC. Finally it was happening.

Tom Allen's story continues in Chapter 12 on p.157.

8

The Impact of Policy Tensions and Organizational Demands on the Process of Moving Out of an Institution

Christine Bigby, Australia

Institutions have been closed and residents moved to small group homes to try and ensure that people with intellectual disabilities are included in the community, have more friends and have more choices. But living in a group home has not always led to these outcomes. This chapter is based on a study in Australia that looked at how 58 people were moved from an institution to live in small group homes. We looked at how the move was organized to try and understand why it did not have all the good outcomes expected. The government decided it would provide the funding for group homes but invited non-government organizations to run the group homes. Staff in the new group homes did not know the residents very well before they moved and could not ask institutional staff about them. There was a lot of information about the residents that staff in the new houses did not know and sometimes the information they were given was wrong. For some people this meant they were not understood by staff, or staff did not help them stay in touch with their friends or family. The organizations had a contract to run the homes for the government but the tasks that staff had to do did not match the aims in the contracts. For example, staff spent most time on cooking and cleaning and caring for people rather than helping them to make choices or make new friends. The contracts said residents should be included in the community but did not provide funds for work to make the community more accepting of people with disabilities. The organizations able to run the group homes had to be large and this meant the senior managers had to know about lots of different groups of people and did not really understand the needs of people with intellectual disabilities very well. Finally, the model of group homes did not give people with disabilities the choice to live in other types of housing arrangements.

In the last three decades, policies of institutional closure and relocation to community living have been used to pursue visions of full citizenship and to realize rights to choice, inclusion and participation in society for people with intellectual disabilities. In the State of Victoria, Australia, between 1976 and 2000, the number of people with intellectual disabilities living in institutions reduced from 4439 to 873 (Bigby, Frederico and Cooper 2004). This was due to the closure of four institutions, the reduction in size of others through relocation of residents to the community and a policy of no new admissions. The dominant model to replace institutional living has been small group homes of four or five residents located in ordinary residential streets.

Meta analyses of the outcomes of relocation to community living for people with intellectual disabilities clearly demonstrate an increased quality of life on a range of dimensions (Emerson and Hatton 1996; Young *et al.* 1998). However, it is also clear from these studies that little change has occurred in relation to the social connectedness and community inclusion of relocated residents. The failure of 'moving out' to deliver the expected outcomes has fuelled debate as to the viability of small-group community living for all people with intellectual disabilities, and led to suggestions that village or cluster-style congregate living may be more desirable (Bigby 2004; Cummins and Lau 2003; Emerson 2004).

An alternative perspective is that the failure may be related to the broader policy context in which the shift from institutional to community care is embedded. The last 20 years have seen the restructuring of welfare states, characterized by an ideological shift to reliance on markets, and reduced collective commitments to vulnerable populations (Esping-Anderson 1996; Ife 1997). Deinstitutionalization and a shift from standard to more flexible services were identified as one of the key changed features of aged and disability services in the European welfare states (Baldock and Evers 1991). Other relevant factors were the more explicit acknowledgement of informal care systems, a shift from bureaucratic centralism to regulated pluralism and the integration of economic with social criteria in service development. The failures of the shift from institutional to community care might stem from difficulties encountered in policy implementation, created by tensions that arise from these broader social policy imperatives of the restructured welfare states. These include, particularly, tensions between economic and social criteria, and the impact of the new policy directions in shaping the utilization of resources during closure processes.

Using findings from a study of the relocation of residents from an institution to the community, this chapter highlights some of the tensions implicit in the relocation process that stem from the social policy imperatives that formed the context and shaped the process. The chapter identifies and discusses factors that contribute to the shortfall in resident outcomes, and contributes to an understanding of issues that must be considered in the ongoing relocation of residents and eventual closure of this and the other remaining institutions in Australia.

Background

This chapter draws on a study of 58 residents relocated from a large institution in Australia to small group homes between 1999 and 2000 (Bigby *et al.* 2004). As is the case with other research, improvements to the residents' overall quality of life after 12 months were found. Many, but not all, residents were judged by others to be happier living in the community, the fabric of their everyday environment was of much higher quality and they lived with more personal space and privacy. However, although use of community facilities increased, few residents participated in any community-based organizations, had established new friendships or acquaintances in their local areas or communities of interest, or had friends or advocates who were not family or paid workers. Residents' choice, autonomy and activities were limited by their membership of a household group, and most spent their weekdays in large groups of people with disabilities in day activity or supported employment programmes.

The findings discussed here are drawn from data about the process of relocation. Organizational and individual planning documents were examined and a focus group held with the team responsible for the relocation. Semi-structured interviews were conducted with various institutional chief executive officers during the period and with the managers from the six non-government organizations responsible for managing the 11 group homes to which residents were relocated. These interviews acquired data about these organizations and the management of the homes. A phone survey of house supervisors sought data about the implementation of the recommendations made by the relocation team. In-depth qualitative case studies of 11 residents from four homes were undertaken during their first year in the community. Descriptive data were analysed thematically, and some open-ended questions in the interview schedules and telephone survey were categorized and descriptive statistics used in their analysis.

Shifting responsibility from the State

A key decision, taken at a senior government level, that community-based services for relocated residents would be competitively tendered and contracted to the non-government sector, set the parameters for the relocation project. Another key decision was that the programme model was to be a five-bedroom group house.

A relocation team within the institution but separate from its day-to-day operations managed the relocation process. The team was responsible for the selection of residents from amongst those who expressed an interest in moving, which occurred in tandem with determining house groupings of residents. Criteria used in selection included individual needs, compatibility, representativeness of the general institutional population (i.e. gender ratio, support-need level) and ability to meet needs within available resources. The model required residents with similar support needs to be grouped together, a decision which gave preference to and at times cut across potential friendship groupings. The relocation team classified the overall support needs of each grouping of residents as high, medium or low, and organizations were invited to submit tenders based on pen portraits of the five proposed residents. All the homes were purpose built and owned by a state government agency which oversaw the building in liaison with the relocation team.

The organizations eventually contracted to manage the group homes were not involved in the costings of support or assessment of residents, and they all reported that oversights and underestimates in these meant much time was consumed in protracted negotiations for additional resources with the contract managers in different administrative regions. They had varying success in negotiations which led to both flexibility and inequalities. For example, two houses managed by one organization argued similar cases for additional funding, successfully in one region but not in another.

Six not-for-profit organizations won the tenders to manage the 11 houses, with five organizations managing more than one house. The organizational mission statements portrayed similar values, using words such as 'well-being' and 'rights', and phrases such as 'to provide effective responses that respectfully support and empower those who are the most disadvantaged and to challenge the social systems that oppress or devalue them' (Bigby *et al.* 2004).

The decision to tender out services reflected a central characteristic of the restructured welfare state, that of shifting the responsibility of the State from funding and service delivery (purchaser and provider) to funding alone. It also reflected the move to apply business principles to the delivery of welfare, and increased marketization through the use of competitive tendering. To achieve these shifts successfully, industrial obstacles have to be overcome, which in this case required the avoidance of the suggestion of 'transmission of business'[1] and the associated financial implications. Various strategies were employed to reinforce the difference between the work of institutional and community-based staff, which together meant the exclusion of institutional staff from the relocation process and emphasized the separation of the relocation team from direct-care staff. The relocation team acted as a 'go-between' and no contact occurred between staff from the organizations responsible for the group homes and institutional direct-care staff.

Information transfer

Due to the separation of roles, organizations and their new staff relied on the documents prepared by the relocation team for information about their new residents. For each resident a report was compiled summarizing his or her background and current circumstances, and recommendations were given for action, and given to the organization together with specialist reports and administrative items, such as taxi card, a month prior to the move. Community staff perceived that the inability to discuss residents with institutional staff and the poor quality of the written reports, which lacked detail, hindered their full understanding of residents, particularly in relation to challenging behaviours and successful strategies for containing them. For example, if upset, one resident had always wandered around the grounds of the institution, yet this was not included in her history. The accuracy of information was criticized and reports were thought to present an overly positive view of some residents to avoid 'scaring off' service providers. One manager said: 'it looked beautiful but it was not a good picture of needs, it lacked the nitty gritty of residents' particular care issues.'

Written medical information was identified as particularly problematic, with an absence of detailed medical histories and information about current diagnosis and treatments. An example of the consequences of this was that when a resident contracted chicken pox, she and the other four residents were confined to the house for two weeks as no one knew which of them had already had this disease. An example of inaccurate information was the discovery that it was another resident rather than the one the reports suggested who was incontinent at night. Several instances occurred where medical check-ups following relocation identified conditions about which no information had been provided at all. For example, one resident, who continually bumped into things, was found to have cataracts in both eyes.

Staff also gave examples of missing information about residents' sexuality and sexual relationships, particularly those of a homosexual nature. In one instance, information about the break-up of a resident's long-term relationship and his subsequent multiple sexual relations with others was not mentioned until emotional issues emerged following the move.

Information dissemination

Problems with the quality of information were compounded by the failure of dissemination and its effective use. Six of the eleven house supervisors were unaware that the written relocation reports included specific recommendations about each resident, and several more did not know either that the reports existed or where they might be found. Instances were found of house staff being unaware of the particular friendships or family constellation of residents, despite these being clearly documented in the relocation report.

After 12 months in the community, 67 per cent of all recommendations made in reports about residents had been acted upon, 15 per cent had been acted upon partially and 18 per cent not at all. In one instance, a resident had not seen his brother who continued to live in the institution due to the failure to implement recommendations which were compounded by staff ignorance of the brother's existence. Another resident did not attend a dance programme in which he had participated for many years as a result of staff knowing neither about his previous attendance nor the recommendation that he continue to attend.

The imperatives of contracting out that drove the process of information transfer impacted on its mode, quality and dissemination. It meant heavy reliance was placed on written rather than more informal avenues of communication between institutional and community-based staff. Use of the formal mode may account for the limited information about sexuality which, though known to staff, was not captured in written reports. This demonstrates the difficulty of applying principles derived from the business world to human services. Capturing and transferring an individual's biography and an accurate picture of their social relationships and health issues is a complex task requiring investigation of different sources and use of various communication modes. It is not similar to writing a product specification. The findings demonstrate the tremendous impact of inaccurate or missing information on residents' social networks, health and well-being, and suggest that multiple modes of information collection are necessary to ensure all aspects of a resident's background are transferred to community staff. Also demonstrated is the need for more active dissemination strategies to front-line staff. Where the information is just not available to be transferred, as was the case with medical histories, proactive strategies prior to relocation are necessary, such as the conduct of professional file reviews, comprehensive medical examination, preparation of summary reports for use by community-based staff and perhaps even briefings with new general practitioners.

Tender and contract specifications

The business rules used by government require that tendering is conducted with probity and very formal specification in contracts of what it is that is to be purchased. In this study the timing and nature of the tendering processes meant successful organizations were excluded from involvement in the design and construction of group homes, and thus their expertise was lost in this phase. This may have contributed to some of the poor designs commented upon by staff. Complaints were made about the physical design of houses, such as the absence of a front fence to ensure resident safety and a bathroom that was too small to fit a needed hoist. In addition, recommendations made by the relocation team about kitchen design were only fully implemented for six of the ten residents for whom they were made. This particularly affected wheelchair users who could not use kitchen benches and sinks. The failure to adapt designs to individual residents may also stem from the economic imperatives that created tensions between a house being regarded as the 'home' of particular residents or simply a generic addition to housing stock, suitable for current and future residents.

Prior to the move, at least three visits were planned for residents to see the new house and meet both staff and other residents. Organizations were funded approximately a month prior to the move to enable this to occur as well as to orientate staff. However, the contracting process is focused on outcome and not inputs. Each organization, free to make its own decisions about the hiring of staff and use of time, took a different approach. For example, one appointed a person to oversee two homes and did not employ any other staff until just prior to the residents' moving, which meant staff did not meet residents until the day of the move. Some moves, including the one mentioned above, were described as chaotic; one house supervisor saw it as:

> a complete mess with the residents running around like 'headless chooks'. The guys arrived in the afternoon, staff had not met them before nor seen where they had been living. Staff felt very ill prepared. They didn't know where to start particularly with washing and toileting.

Building delays meant the last phase of transition was often rushed, and in at least one instance residents moved a week after their first visit. Their home, like several others, was not fully finished or furnished and, in the absence of a dining table and chairs, they sat on the floor to eat for the first few nights.

The nature of contracts between the government and non-government organizations and the consequent financial considerations contributed to the rushed and sometimes chaotic moves to incomplete houses. This was exacerbated by the necessity to match the timing of residents' moves with the closure of specific units and redeployment of staff and residents within the institution. The contingencies resting on a set date for moving were too many and complex to warrant a delay. Factors such as this mean the centrality of resident well-being to relocation processes is lost, thus compromising optimal outcomes for residents.

Difficulties also occurred because of a purchaser–provider split and a hands-off 'business' relationship between government and non-government organizations. Whilst the aims of community inclusion were specified, implementation and inputs in this regard were left to the contracted organization. Rather than increasing the prescription of service models, as suggested by Felce and his colleagues (1998) as necessary to take account of the knowledge required and complexity of policy implementation, marketization has reduced it. The evidence suggests a failure to effectively translate these aims into day-to-day practices within the houses. For example, the job descriptions of house supervisors and other staff conveyed expectations of providing inclusion and developmental opportunities for residents as well as day-to-day care. For example, one job description stated the aim as: 'To offer the residents a valued place in society through high quality care and opportunities to participate in the community and interact with its members.' Detailed position duties, however, focused more on domestic management and care, including attention to financial matters of the house and residents, documentation and administration, cooking and cleaning. Tasks such as this outnumbered those associated with development of social relationships or inclusion. In one organization only 6 of the 24 tasks specified in the job description required direct interaction with residents. Data from the intensive case studies showed that staff spent most of their time providing day-to-day care and that daily routines were organized around getting things done rather than resident engagement in the running of the household. One staff member said: 'Just getting through every day and feeling that you have given each resident a bit of time, and everybody is happy, as to achieving anything else, it doesn't happen.'

Attention was drawn by supervisors to the difficulties of implementing individual programme plans, with confusion about with whom and with which programme, day or residential, responsibility for implementation lay. No one had ongoing formal responsibility to mediate between staff from different programmes or to take a broader long-term planning perspective in a resident's life. One staff member commented:

> The problem is that you don't know what the other staff are doing or how they are behaving. There is no chance to implement programmes as there is no one to work with and no consistency. It's hard enough doing the basics, the everyday things.

House supervisors received little support from more senior personnel in their organizations when it came to planning for the development of social relationships or community participation. They also had responsibility to identify local medical and allied health practitioners, a task for which they felt ill equipped. They reported taking residents to doctors and other professionals who did not know how to relate to people with intellectual disabilities. Few mechanisms were in place to share knowledge between staff in houses in the same locality, and many house staff were unfamiliar with the locality of the house and local community resources. Little evidence was found of linkages either between the houses or to their locality after 12 months.

Contract specifications were focused narrowly on the residents for whom the organizations provided care. They were silent on the broader collective context which underpins opportunities for community inclusion of individual residents. A very privatized version of inclusion was built into the contracts, suggesting that contracted organizations bore the sole responsibility for all aspects of community living for residents. This is unrealistic. The broader community development or education functions that relate to whole populations and tackle obstacles – such as community attitudes, resourcing of community facilities for inclusion, and the limited knowledge and skills of staff in the community – are vital to facilitate individual inclusion outcomes.

The danger in a marketized system such as this is that community development tasks unrelated to specific individual outcomes are not specified or purchased, and are left undone as it is not clear with whom such responsibilities lie or where the costs should fall. For example, in this study no action was taken to tackle systemic issues identified by house staff, such as the discriminatory attitudes of taxi drivers and the need to support general practitioners and other heath professionals in relating to people with intellectual disabilities.

Staff in group homes are faced with the complex and multi-faceted task of supporting community inclusion, yet they received little resourcing for this role from the broader organizations for which they worked or through complementary programmes in the community. This project demonstrates the poor outcomes that result from adoption of a single very privatized strategy for achieving inclusion rather than the multiplicity of strategies that have been suggested as necessary (Bigby 1999). It is notable that the current state government, elected after the commencement of this project, while it has not retreated from the contracting out of services, has reframed relationships with the non-government sector to perceive them as partners rather than as businesses or contractors, and placed greater emphasis on collective responsibility for creating conditions for community inclusion through specific funding for community development projects.

Impact of marketization

In Australia, marketization of community services has driven the amalgamation of smaller single-programme local agencies and the formation of larger statewide multi-function organizations. Government policy has also emphasized cross-disability rather than diagnostically based services for people with disabilities. These trends are reflected in the size and nature of the organizations in the study. All had some experience in managing residential services for people with intellectual disabilities, but for most their expertise lay in the physical and sensory disability field. The largest had over 1000 staff and 30 programmes, and the smallest had 170 staff and 5 programmes. They were all state-wide organizations rather than being locally or regionally based. These characteristics are not commensurate with those of organizations identified by Taylor and his colleagues as producing 'best practice' outcomes in this field, which include being of a small size, being focused on particular groups, being decentralized and retaining a hands-on approach by managers (Taylor, Bogdan and Racino 1991). Large generic organizations mean that managers may be unskilled in relation to particular groups for whom they provide services, and make it difficult to model good practice and retain a vision for or strong commitment to particular groups (Mansell 1996).

Standard or flexible models

The model of a five-bedroom group home in the community is less standardized and has significantly greater potential for flexibility than institutional care. It did, however, require residents to be slotted in places, with the primary basis for house groupings being similarity of support needs rather than individual choice or friendship grouping. This criterion was criticized by community staff as leading to inappropriate groups of people with very high support needs. Residents did not have individual tenancy rights or control over who else lived in their home. Ericsson (1996) suggests that models such as this do not separate housing and support, and make it more difficult to achieve a 'citizenship' model, whereby choice is paramount and supports are provided on individual terms.

Funding for daytime support was through the placement of residents into day programmes, which staff suggested contributed to the fragmentation of residents' lives and led to issues of cross-programme communication. It led to rigid daytime routines, with residents having little choice but to attend a full-time day programme. Funds could not be used flexibly to enable residents to remain at home or purchase more intensive individual activities for shorter periods. The necessity of travelling to day centres in other communities did not foster inclusion in the locality of their home and meant residents often incurred significant daily travel costs.

The adoption of a uniform model of group community-living support for all residents represents only partial progress along the continuum of flexibility. It suggests that economic criteria may have been the overriding factor in the relocation and that this detracted from individual resident choice, flexibility and the centrality of outcomes for residents. More flexible approaches that foster ongoing choice and opportunities for spontaneity are found in individualized consumer-directed models of funding support that are now being adopted as the preferred model for new funding by various state government disability programmes in Australia (Bigby 1999).

Summary

This chapter has described the processes of moving 58 people from a large institution to small groups living in the community. It identifies some of the factors that impact on achieving optimal outcomes for residents and create obstacles to the maintenance and formation of social relationships, participation and inclusion in local communities. The chapter has argued that the policies of deinstitutionalization can be confounded by the tensions created by the broader social policy context in which disability policy is situated. Such tensions vary over time and with the complexion of governments. But making them explicit at least provides opportunities to understand why some of the unrealized expectations for moving out occur, and may enable us to confront the obstacles rather than retreat back to the safety of segregated living for people with intellectual disabilities. This chapter also suggests that the disability field must recognize and become a key player in broader social policy developments that shape possibilities for the effective implementation of disability policy. Community inclusion cannot be the responsibility of disability services alone and will not be achieved by individual privatized measures. It is a responsibility that requires action from whole communities and across all parts of government administrations.

Note

1 The concept of transmission of business requires the government to demonstrate that the same business is not simply being transferred to the non-government sector, where pay and conditions are poorer than in the government sector. If this simple transmission is demonstrated, then industrial agreements require that pay and conditions from the government sector also be transferred.

References

Baldock, J. and Evers, A. (1991) 'Innovations and care of the elderly: The frontline of change in social welfare services.' *Ageing International*, June, 8–21.

Bigby, C. (1999) 'International trends.' In E. Ozanne, C. Bigby, S. Forbes, C. Glennen, M. Gordon and C. Fyffe: *Reframing Opportunities for People with an Intellectual Disability*. A report funded by the Myer Foundation. Melbourne: University of Melbourne.

Bigby, C. (2004) 'But why are these questions being asked? Invited opinions and perspectives.' *Journal of Intellectual and Developmental Disabilities 29*, 3, 202–205.

Bigby, C., Frederico., M. and Cooper, B. (2004) *Not just a Residential Move but Creating a Better Lifestyle for People with Intellectual Disabilities: Report of the Evaluation of Kew Residential Services Community Relocation Project 1999.* Melbourne: Department of Human Services.

Cummins, R. and Lau, A. (2003) 'Community integration or community exposure? A review and discussion in relation to people with an intellectual disability.' *Journal of Applied Research in Intellectual Disability 16*, 145–57.

Emerson, E. (2004) 'Cluster housing for adults with intellectual disabilities.' *Journal of Intellectual and Developmental Disabilities 29*, 3, 187–97.

Emerson, E. and Hatton, C. (1996) 'Deinstitutionalisation in the UK and Ireland: Outcomes for service users.' *Journal of Intellectual and Developmental Disabilities 21*, 1, 17–37.

Ericsson, K. (1996) 'Housing for the person with intellectual disability.' In J. Mansell and K. Ericsson (eds) *Deinstitutionalisation and Community Living: Intellectual Disability Services in Britain, Scandinavia and United States.* London: Chapman and Hall.

Esping-Andersen, G. (1996) *Welfare States in Transition: National Adaptations to Global Economies.* London: Sage Publications in association with United Nations Institute for Social Development.

Felce, D., Grant, G., Todd, S., Ramcharan, P., Beyer, S., McGrath, M., Perry, J., Shearn, J., Kilsby, M. and Lowe, K. (1998) *Towards a Full Life: Researching Policy Innovation for People with Learning Disabilities.* Oxford: Butterworth Heinemann.

Ife, J. (1997) *Rethinking Social Work: Towards Critical Practice.* Melbourne: Longman.

Mansell, J. (1996) 'Issues in community services in Britain.' In J. Mansell and K. Ericsson (eds) *Deinstitutionalisation and Community Living: Intellectual Disability Services in Britain, Scandinavia and United States.* London: Chapman and Hall.

Taylor, S., Bogdan, R. and Racino, J. (1991) *Life in the Community: Case Studies of Organisations Supporting People with Disabilities.* Baltimore, MD: Paul H. Brookes.

Young, L., Sigafoos, J., Suttie, J. and Ashman, A. (1998) 'Deinstitutionalisation of persons with intellectual disabilities: A review of Australian studies.' *Journal of Intellectual and Developmental Disabilities 23*, 2, 155–70.

9

The Cost of Moving Out

Ingiborg Eide Geirsdóttir
with Gudrún V. Stefánsdóttir, Iceland

I grew up in a small fishing village. Our house was on a hill by the sea and I could see the tide come in. I lived with my father and mother, my two sisters and brother. I could not walk well till I was seven years old. I could not run around and play with the other children, and that made me angry and sad. I went to school in the village when I was seven. I was there for two years. The headmaster told my mother there was an institution in the south and said I should go there. When I was a little girl nobody said I was retarded. I just had twisted legs. But in the institution everybody was retarded and so was I. That is strange.

I remember well when I went to the institution in 1959. I was nine years old. It was difficult to move away from my family. I wanted to stay with them. I was often angry when I lived in the institution. Sometimes I hit people and then I was locked in my room.

There were many of us girls in the same room; the beds were side by side and I had to crawl over other beds to get into mine. I did a lot of work in the institution and so did all the other girls. We had plays at Christmas, and Independence Day was fun.

My brother and sisters helped me move into the first group home that was established in Reykjavík. But in order to move there I had to be sterilized. I was not happy about that at first but then I agreed. Once I wanted to have a child but no longer. They also operated on all the other women who lived in the group home. We were all sterilized.

I moved into the group home in 1976. I was 26. It was good to move away from the institution but there were too many people living in the group home. It was difficult to live with so many people. Now I have my own flat. I have lived here since 1993. Now I can do what I want. That is good. I like to write poems and I work in the hospital laundry. I have worked there more than 20 years. I like the work and the people I work with. I have many friends and I often see my family. I have a good life now.

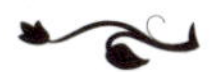

Gudrún writes: This story is based on interviews with Ingiborg Eide Geirsdóttir, her brother and sisters, and some of the people who have worked closely with her. These interviews were tape-recorded and transcribed. After each interview with Ingiborg, I read the transcripts for her and she added new information. Based on these interview transcripts, Ingiborg's life story has been constructed in close co-operation with her and, for the most part, in her own words. The story below is a small part of a much longer and more detailed story of Ingiborg's life.

Ingiborg was born in 1950 in a small fishing village in Iceland. She has two sisters and one brother who are close to her in age. Ingiborg lived in the village until she was nine years old when she was sent to live in an institution for people with intellectual disabilities in a different part of Iceland, far away from her family. She lived in the institution for 17 years. For much of that time she had limited contact with her family. Her mother visited her once a year, but when her brother and sisters became adults they re-established contact with Ingiborg and now she has very close ties with her siblings.

In 1976, at the age of 26, Ingiborg moved to the first group home for people with intellectual disabilities that was established in Reykjavík, the capital of Iceland. Her siblings applied for her to be allowed to live in the group home.

During the application process it was made clear to them that Ingiborg would not be allowed to move out of the institution and into the group home unless she was sterilized. Her siblings found this very difficult to accept, but there was no choice. If Ingiborg was to leave the institution she had to be sterilized. Reluctantly they agreed and undertook to obtain Ingiborg's consent. According to Ingiborg, all the other women who moved into the group home also had to undergo sterilization in order to live there.

Ingiborg's story

Childhood at home

My father was a labourer and worked at the harbour. My mother didn't work outside our home but instead took care of our home and us children, and she also had to buy the food. In the mornings I always got porridge and sausage, and at noon fish and potatoes, and then we drank water at mealtimes. For afternoon 'coffee' we had bread and milk, and in the evening my mother cooked soup and often gave us bread with it. It isn't really healthy to eat two hot meals a day. They raised me, my mother and my father.

The house we lived in was on a hill by the sea and I could look out and see the tide come in and the shore when the tide went out. I played on the shore. In the evenings my father read to me and my brother and sisters. He also often told me stories and talked to me. My mother was usually cooking and tending to us four children.

I couldn't walk well until I was seven. I had to wear leg braces and I couldn't run after my sisters and that made me mad. My sisters and the other kids in the village often played 'giant steps' and other games I couldn't play. I was sad that I couldn't do what my sisters did. I was also often tied down because it was very steep down to the shore from our house. So I had to watch as the other kids played and I couldn't play with them. That made me mad.

I went to school in the village when I was seven. I was there for two years. My sister always went with me to school and waited for me. I don't remember much about the school but the headmaster told my mother that there was an institution in the south and that I should go there. When I was a little girl nobody said that I was retarded. I just had twisted legs. But in the institution everybody was retarded and so was I. That seems strange to me.

I remember very well when I was moved to the institution in the south: 4 September 1959. I was only nine when I was sent there and I shall never forget it. I went by plane. A woman named Jóna went with me. She lived in the village. Then dad's brother drove me to the institution. It felt strange. I remember it well. I had two suitcases with my clothes. It was no fun to move south away from my father and mother and my brother and sisters. I only wanted to stay with them.

In the institution

In the institution I always had to make my bed and sweep and scrub the floors with all the other girls. Then we always wore our best clothes on Sundays and I still do. The clothes were hung on hangers and I always put them on the hangers very carefully. Then we all had baths on Tuesdays and Fridays. Those were bath days. Now I have a bath every day but the first years I lived in the group home I used to take a bath on Tuesday and Friday, just like in the institution. There were many of us girls in the same room. The beds were side by side and I had to crawl over Bagga's bed to get to mine.

I was often angry when I lived in the institution. Now I think it was because I wanted to be with my father and mother and my brother and sisters. Sometimes I hit the people who worked there and then I was locked in my room. Sometimes for a short time. Sometimes for a long time. I didn't like that, it was no fun.

I learned handicrafts when I was a kid. There was a woman who taught me to sew, knit and crochet. I learned to read when I was 17 years old.

Independence Day was always fun. Everybody was dressed up. Lots of people came and my brother always came with his boy and we marched in the parade. Later my sisters came too and their children. Then coffee and refreshments were served in the institution: flat bread with smoked lamb, cakes and cream, and meringue cakes.

When I was little I was at the institution every Christmas. I wanted to be with my mother and father and my sisters and brother at Christmas time. We always got Christmas presents and we had a play about the birth of Jesus and other stories from the Bible. I was often the Virgin Mary, but I once played a shepherd and once one of the Wise Men. There were all kinds of decorations. Before Christmas, on 21 December, men from the American military base came and gave all the children Christmas gifts. I was grown up by then and did not need these gifts but all the children in the institution were happy to get toys for Christmas.

The summer of 1972 I went home to the village to visit my mother. My father had died before that. He had a brain tumour and died suddenly. I don't think he felt much pain. He died when I was 12.

I went in a big plane to visit my mother. The director of the institution drove me to the airport and some men drove me home to the village. One of them asked me if I knew the way home. Of course I knew the way home! My mother met me at the door and helped me with my suitcases. So the next day my brother came and my sister-in-law and they slept up in the loft. I couldn't sleep. My brother had to drive me back to the big plane to Reykjavík because I couldn't sleep. I had to get back to my own bed in the south.

My brother and sisters often visited me after they moved to Reykjavík. By then I was 15 years old. After that I was always with them for Christmas and also for Easter and often in the summer. I also visited my sister when she lived in the country. My mother visited me at the institution when she was in town. After she moved to an old people's home in the south, she often came to visit me.

On the first Saturday of every month I take the bus to visit the institution. I think it is really strange that people there are always given a ration of cookies and coffee, and Heida and Sigga cannot decide for themselves what they can offer me. They can't even decide for themselves how many cookies they can have. Staff members also do all the cooking and Heida and Sigga are not allowed to. I find it strange that Heida still lives in the institution where everything is rationed. It is shameful not to let people in the institution put cookies in a bowl and let them choose for themselves what they want. When I lived there it was like that too. I find it tiring, no fun. I always want to do things for myself.

The group homes

My brother and sisters learned that a group home for disabled people had been established and told me about it. I wanted to move there. My brother told me that the people in the institution had not wanted me to move to the group home because I was so good at helping out in the institution. I have always been able to help and I want everything around me to be clean and fine and everything in its place.

When I moved to the group home I had to be sterilized. I wasn't happy about that at first, but I agreed. Once I wanted to have a child but no longer. They also operated on all the other women who lived in that group home. We were all sterilized. I was operated on in the gynaecological ward of the hospital. I remember well that I went to the hospital on Wednesday and the operation was on Thursday. Then on Friday my sister came to get me and I stayed with her for a whole week. Then on Saturday I went to a masked ball as a baker. That seemed strange to me. I used to think about this a lot, the sterilization, and it made me angry. But not any more.

I moved to the group home on 21 August 1976. I remember it well. I went on Friday to a furniture store to buy furniture, as I could not be without furniture. My brother and my sisters went in the car with me. They drove with the furniture, the bureau and chair and bed and baskets I had bought. When I turned 40 my brother and sisters gave me a bookcase. I enjoy reading and I have lots of books and I read every evening before I go to bed.

During the first years in the group home I lived in a big bedroom on the top floor. There were others who were in the other rooms and we all ate together and took turns cooking. I found it difficult to live with so many people. There were seven of us. I wasn't allowed to have much say about how things were managed. I often got mad when someone forgot to shut the door or forgot to shut a drawer in the cupboard. I want to decide for myself how things are. It bothers me if things are not where they should be.

Then in 1984 I moved to another group home. There were six of us who lived there. Svanhvít, she lived on the second floor. She is dead now. She got a tumour in the abdomen in October 1994 and then she just died in November. I thought that was a great pity. She was an awfully good woman. I'll never forget how she teased me. I thought that was great fun. We were good friends.

Örn, he lived there too. We are good friends and he sometimes comes to have coffee with me. I like Örn a lot. Sometimes I take him with me to be with my family at my sister's. I also always invite him for my birthday.

I also had a friend named Hördur but he is dead now. He was hit by a car and died. He gave me a pretty picture that hangs in my living room. I often asked him over for coffee and then I baked my special coffee bread. We went to the cinema, too. We had a lot of fun together and he teased me and told me jokes. Then we laughed a great deal. I thought it was too bad that he was hit by a car and died.

My own flat

I moved into the basement of the group home on 30 October 1993 and have been there ever since in my own flat. Then I bought a big dining-room table and my brother gave me a white shelf. Now I live alone and can do what I want. I cook for myself and sometimes get help with it. I also have food in the freezer. On Tuesdays and Fridays I go shopping to buy food. I have my own money that I work for and I go to the bank myself. I can always ring up my sister.

I always wake up at half past seven in the morning and then I eat breakfast and then go to work. When I get home from work I always have afternoon coffee and then I write poems. I began to write poems when I was 21. In the drawer under my bed I have lots of poems I have written in exercise books. Once a poem I wrote was published in the paper. After I have written poems I take a bath at five o'clock. At quarter to six I start thinking about supper and I always eat at six o'clock. After supper I watch TV and have a glass of tea and fruit. I go to bed at ten. Of course, I stay up later when I go to a party. Sometimes I go to the cinema and the theatre with my friend.

Work

I work in the hospital laundry. I began working there on 7 October 1974. At that time I was living in the institution. I always went to work by bus and now I take city bus no. 9. At first I worked all day but now I work only from 9am until 1.30pm. When I was in the institution I got only 2000 kronur a month but that was because I was paid by the day. I had to pay for the bus and lunch at noon. Now I get paid much more.

I have always counted the pieces of laundry in the plastic bags. There should be 50 in each bag. There are lots of foreign women who work with me. They speak another language and they are not always understandable, even when they are speaking Icelandic.

I have worked with the same woman for many years. I like her. She is a good woman. She always hangs up her smock on a hanger. Then she lets the machine fold the laundry. Her husband also works in the laundry. He works with the dirty laundry and sorts it and always has to wear rubber gloves. Their daughter goes to school, she always starts at eight in the morning. I invited them all to my fiftieth birthday but they couldn't come. The woman's friend also had a birthday on 7 October and invited her to her birthday too. I thought that was all right. So many people came to my birthday party, both women and men. I had it at my sister's house.

There's a good canteen where I work, which always has good food. I always eat hot food there. I also meet people there who work in the laundry and I think it's fun talking to them. I have always liked my work. My feet get a little tired sometimes because I have to stand so much. But overall my life is good.

10

Rowan's Choices

Ethel M. Temby, Australia

Rowan is my son. He was born with an intellectual disability. Soon after he was born his father and I were told by doctors that he should live in an institution and that we should not visit him. At first we obeyed their instructions but then I started visiting him with his brothers and sisters. Institutionalization was what happened to most people with intellectual disabilities. He made some friends there and some of the staff were great. He also had some bad times there. Gradually we came to the view that he should come home to live and go to a day centre. Rowan did this when he was 14 and had to learn to make choices for himself. Some of the choices he learned were choosing things to eat, choosing to be caring of others and not to take their things, and choosing to act his age rather than behave like a little boy. He also learned how to cross the road safely and to do jobs around the house. When he was a little older he began to go to a special school. This was important for him.

But when Rowan left school he was bored at home with nothing to do. We found out about a community where there were great relationships between staff and the people with intellectual disabilities who lived there and where there were exciting things to do. Rowan went to live there and loved it. He worked in the bakery, went to plays and concerts and performed in them too. He enjoyed bush walking and went on bike rides and excursions. But gradually the good ideas of the community died away and the people who believed in them left. It was time to move on.

Rowan now lives in an ordinary house with three of his friends. He has just moved in and he chose the people he wanted to live with. A new choice has been made and a new stage of his life has begun.

Rowan's story

Rowan's first fourteen years

Rowan was born in July 1957. When I was discharged from hospital we were told that Rowan would need to remain, because of a collapsed lung condition. We had no choice. When Rowan was a month old our doctor visited Alan and me and brought a paediatrician with him. Two minutes into the visit, they said: 'We have done further tests and find that your baby is mentally retarded.' Stunned, with a sense that my body had gone and my head had become the size of an orange, I asked: 'What does that mean?' The reply was: 'He'll appreciate food and warmth, very little else. He'll really be just a blob.'

They then said: 'You must make up your own minds, of course, but in our opinion you should put him in the Kew Cottages [an institution for people with an intellectual disability] and forget him. Never visit him again.' They valued him at nothing. He was our baby. Traumatized, totally inexperienced and ignorant, we of course had no basis for choice. Besides, in those days everyone believed that what the doctor told us was medical advice. It was some time before it began to dawn on me that what they expressed that night was simply the folklore of the time when a baby with an intellectual disability was born. We didn't visit Rowan and I felt I had murdered him by neglect. Six weeks later they rang and said he was very ill. He had pneumonia. We went to see him. In charge of that cottage was a refugee infant welfare nurse from a Baltic country, an outstanding woman.

After that night I was at Kew about four times a week, both during and after school times, so that Rowan's sister and four brothers knew him and became familiar with the other babies, toddlers and older people in the institution. Their perceptions also were rapidly expanding. These visits started the unending road of changing the attitudes and practices that stemmed from misconceptions of who Rowan was, and led later to his making all the significant choices in his life.

So Rowan grew up with the same staff and the same children until he was six, and we were still pleased with his environment. That winter I had five sick children at home and couldn't get over to Kew to visit Rowan or take him out in the car to pick the others up from school. When I was able to visit him, I was told he wasn't there any more! Unknown to us, he, alone of all the children in that cottage, had been taken to a part of the institution he had never seen before, with no little girls, and to staff who were strangers. He was one among 33 other boys already living there. He had been moved because he was becoming mischievous. They should instead have celebrated this!

I was pleased to find that the woman in charge there was another Baltic refugee whose background was in preschool education. She told me he had fretted for three days before she had been able to get the assistance of a young woman who had worked in the cottage up the hill and was well known to Rowan. Rowan's ability for self-expression is very limited, but his fretting indicated his preferences to a sensitive woman. This was a major emotional trauma for Rowan.

In 1968, when Rowan was ten, the Australian parents of children with intellectual disabilities and government invited Doctor Rosemary and Professor Gunnar Dybwad to visit as counsellors. The Dybwads' visit was extremely significant. Hearing them, it became totally clear to us that Rowan must be given the opportunity to live at home and attend a day centre.

Rowan at home

When Rowan was 14 we were suddenly offered a day place at a school for children with a moderate disability, and Rowan came home on 'trial leave' the next day. To prevent the traumas he had twice endured at Kew, and which I believe still affect him, we arranged for him to be home during the week and to return to Kew at weekends. For five weeks he was pleased with this, but on the sixth Friday when I told him it was the day Dad would take him 'to see Wally and the boys', he would not put his clothes on after school. When I eventually explained that it would be kind to go over and say goodbye, and that if he wanted to do that he would be able to stay at home all the time, he put out his hand for the clothes. He had made a very significant lifestyle choice. To me it was also wonderful that he chose kindness.

Rowan came from Kew at 14 with the social behaviour of a toddler. No one in that environment had ever expected the residents to need to learn about traffic hazards, behaviour suitable to age, consideration for others' possessions, and so on. We soon realized also that the institution never allowed choice. When Rowan came home to live he was incapable of even choosing a biscuit from a plate, let alone a spare-time activity or which clothes to wear, or even when to get a drink of water. His life had been lived for 14 years under total staff direction.

But Rowan chose to learn these things. We bought a loaf of bread. At the shop door Rowan turned and blew kisses to the shopkeeper. When we were outside I told him that little kids did that, and named a couple of small neighbours, but that big boys didn't. 'Does Peter do it?' Shake of head. 'Does Ian?' Shake. 'Does Johnny?' Shake. And so on through the family, then: 'Do you want to?' 'No', and he never did it again. He learnt many things that way, including not taking others' possessions and hiding them under his pillow or mattress. Very difficult choice that one!

Several years later came a splendid outcome of learning to choose. Rowan loved helping one of our neighbours who was landscaping his block of land. Harry had just asked Rowan if he'd like to give him a hand, when a telephone message required me to visit my sister at once. 'Rowan, would you like to come to Auntie Ol's or stay and help Harry?' No answer. 'Rowan, do you want to stay with Harry?' 'Yes.' 'Do you want to come to see Auntie Ol?' 'Not yet.' Harry and I looked at each other with delight and then we laughed and Rowan stayed with Harry. He had not only made a choice but he had made clear that he reserved a second choice. Good on him.

Rowan loved the day school and the family environment, but he started wandering off without saying anything. Many times this happened and the anxiety was awful. Finally I told him that if he kept going away I would have to take him back to Kew. He continued, so I told him to get into the car and I drove to Kew, parking very near the ward he had lived in before he came home. He refused to get out and locked the car door so I couldn't open it. Great initiative, but maddening!

Back inside the car, I told him yet again how frightened I was when I couldn't find him or if he didn't answer when I called him. I told him it made me feel sick and very worried, because I didn't know whether he was hurt or had fallen into the river, and that was why I'd brought him back to Kew. To my delight and amazement he said: 'Sorry, Mum.' And his were not the only tear-filled eyes.

That day Rowan made the choice of living in the ordinary family environment with all its demands: rough and tumbles with older brothers, and coping with neighbours, a shop and a bus to catch for school. And he was lucky to have one particularly perceptive teacher who, after a year, sent home a note to say: 'Today Rowan printed his name and the tears ran down his face into his grin.'

Almost three years later, on a hot December day, there was a picnic at the day centre with families and their children from another part of Melbourne. Through the afternoon I noticed Rowan playing a group game with six or seven others. Then I sat up when I realized that none of them were his schoolmates. They were all children from the visiting families and all much, much brighter than he was. So I got the message that perhaps he was out of his context at that school.

That night I applied for him to move to a government school supposedly banned to anyone with a severe disability. After the expected long delays he was accepted into the nearest special school, where they said he was educationally advantaged and the other children socially advantaged. Wow! And the school was only supposed to take children with a mild disability. That was another of Rowan's choices.

Rowan had been living at home for about a year when the paddocks around us were subdivided and a road was built in front of us. Houses quickly followed and our road, with a curve on the left and a rise on our right, began to have a lot of traffic. The freedom of the paddocks was gone. Rowan needed to learn to cross the roads independently. Asked if he'd like to learn this, he said 'yes', but without any understanding. It was as if he were offered a piece of cake. Well, this piece of cake was about a year in the oven. At first he saw trucks or cars and smiled and said the word as if collecting dinky toys in his head. Certainly not seeing them as dangerous in any way. That took ages.

When I was absolutely certain he knew what he was doing, I asked him if he'd like to take me across the road with my eyes shut. Broad grin and emphatic yes. So I took his hand and shut my eyes, told him to look at my shut eyes and asked him to take me to the other side of the road. No, I didn't cheat. At the other side I stumbled on the kerb and that opened my eyes suddenly. He looked about six inches taller and his grin nearly split the back of his head. A fantastic graduation ceremony. I have never cautioned him since. He owns that responsibility. Unfortunately, few others have respected this.

During these years his father and I had spent a month of 1974 in South Africa for a family wedding. A social worker I met suggested we visit a place in Cape Colony. We had a whole day and were immensely comfortable with the relationships we saw between people with intellectual disabilities, who were living and working there, and their supporters. We were also impressed with the degree of initiative and creativity the supporters encouraged.

In 1978 I attended an international congress in Vienna, and on the day of visits selected what was listed as a preschool centre. Our guide at the centre spent the morning telling us in English, French and Spanish what their philosophy was and what was happening at that school, so I had time to think. At the end of the morning I said, 'This sounds remarkably like the Steiner philosophy', to which he replied: 'Oh yes, this is a Waldorf school.' By then I'd found that the South African place was a Camphill village and we had visited the Steiner boarding school in Victoria. The Steiner place I then visited in Sydney had the same 'feel'.

In three such different political and social environments, it was evident that the strength of the Rudolf Steiner principles of living for people with disabilities remained strong and consistent, regardless of political and social differences.

We were strongly attracted to an environment that not only encouraged and supported ongoing development of all aspects of a person (intellectual, emotional, physical, social, spiritual, etc.) but also positively created a sense of responsibility and caring for others in the community. And that was the key to the ambience of all the Steiner places we had visited. So we put Rowan's name on a waiting list for the Victorian Steiner place, as insurance only.

Like everyone else in the family, Rowan had jobs to do. One was to get me a hod of coke after school for our Aga stove. He liked doing this and demonstrating how strong he was. Then one day when I needed to fuel up the stove before dinner the hod was empty. 'Rowan, you haven't got the coke for me. I need it now, so you go and get it.' No move from Rowan, just a stare. I repeated what I had said. Still no move. Several repetitions later he leant forward and prompted me with 'please'! So I explained that I hadn't said please because it was his job and he hadn't done it, so it was for him to go and do it without a special request from me. He understood and went out the door, banged it and muttered something outside that sounded very like swearing. He had never heard anyone swear in our house, but had chosen when it was appropriate. He had learned at Kew how to swear vigorously in German.

Adult years

Rowan was required by law in our state to leave school before he turned 21. It was July. The adult centre reluctantly accepted him in September. With the loss of the stimulus of school he was bored and started wandering further and further from home, apparently in search of additional interest and activity. Then, out of the blue, we had an invitation in December to visit the Steiner place with Rowan. His father and I spent the afternoon walking and talking and drinking tea with our hostess. Then she said: 'We'd like to invite Rowan to join us.' Not 'We could give him a bed or a place', but an invitation that revealed many qualities. We were not thinking of Rowan leaving home, but accepted a fortnight stay in February, as I would be helping with his sister's toddler while my daughter had another baby.

When we went to pick Rowan up he didn't want to come with us. He had made his choice of a living environment for a second time. So he moved out of home, as is customary with most young adults. He chose to live at a Steiner community at Wandin, where he had previously spent a fortnight.

Rowan came home for holidays and celebrations. At Wandin, a large hilly property, his all-round growth continued and his favourite activity was working in the bakery. Unable to do the arithmetic, he learnt the rhythm of the ingredients to put together for a batch of bread and became an expert in the skill of kneading to make a perfect loaf. The baker referred to him as his 'right-hand man'. His previous experiences in the pottery, the nursery, the vegetable garden gave him nothing of the satisfaction of the bread-making. Offered changes, he rejected them without hesitation. At Wandin, Rowan had many opportunities for creativity – in music groups, in taking part in the seasonal plays – once an adaptation of one of Shakespeare's dramas – in various forms of handiwork, in listening and contributing to stories, in dance or sometimes in going to an evening concert. He also went bush walking, visited a youth hostel on a cycling trip and rode weekly to a swimming pool with two others. There were no 'flock' outings; normality was important. Soon his preference was to stay at Wandin rather than come home.

Evidence of the pain of his unremembered traumas at Kew, when moves had caused misery and loss of friends, showed every time he needed to leave Wandin. But it only took minutes, when he finally got into my car, before he'd say: 'I'm happy, Mum.' This still happens, so I ask staff to tell him days before that I'll be coming to take him, and for what purpose.

However, application of the Steiner training and philosophy fell away over time, and the dilution by staff from other backgrounds gradually changed the emphases and the perceptions of the Wandin environment. Finally, a complete change of management became a necessity. By then no Steiner people remained. The philosophical environment his father and I had sought, and Rowan had chosen, had only intermittent remnants left.

People who had heard about the right to choose often interpreted it superficially and failed to accept the greater human right to be helped to choose with discrimination. It seemed that phrases which, when introduced, had stimulated thought, had through time become no more than clichés. The philosophical focus on supporting the ongoing full development of the person was lost in the practicalities of daily living.

Explanations of Rowan's simple, practical and personal behaviour needs, repeated many times to a frequently changing staff, led nowhere. He regressed in a number of ways. He was usually not given informed choices; he was mostly given 'prompts'.

A return to full community living, with neighbours either side and over the road, became overwhelmingly attractive, provided Rowan could share with his two close friends and their familiar support workers. Rowan had selected his two friends from 28 photos of all residents at Wandin at a meeting of Victoria's Intellectual Disability Review Panel, which advises government. All three of them chose each other.

Two years of advocacy and endless repetitions in many varied ways to numerous recipients within the government bureaucracy finally achieved a move for Rowan with his two friends into a suburban house. From his bedroom window he looks down a front lawn to the street, and clothes dry on a line in the backyard. The three staff who alternate in overnight stays are all of the same mind about personal dignity and importance.

The house has been leased for two years. All of its residents are pleased with the move. They go to different day programmes and plan to dig up part of the back lawn for a vegetable garden. I hope they will offer surplus vegetables to their neighbours. They have just moved in, so though they are in the community they are not yet part of it. If Rowan has anything to do with it, that will soon follow.

11

Moving Out

A Reflection

Kelley Johnson, Australia

For people with intellectual disabilities who have lived in large institutions, moving out into the community is a life-changing event. However, often people are not given information about how decisions are made as to where they will live, with whom they will live or what they will do when they move into the community. The chapters in this part of the book give accounts of some of the different ways people with intellectual disabilities have experienced moving out. Some people, like Tom Allen, went to court to win the right to leave an institution. Others, like Ingiborg, paid a high price for a place in the community: she had to agree to sterilization in order to be allowed to have an apartment. Moving out of an institution can also be a sad time for some people with intellectual disabilities, as they lose contact with friends and places that were important to them. Sometimes family or friends can help with these feelings but there is little counselling offered to people to help them with their feelings at this time.

The chapters in this part of the book show how important it is for people with intellectual disabilities to have family or advocates or friends to support them in moving out. Sometimes this means that families have to change their ideas about 'what is good for' their family member. And sometimes what families want and what the person with a disability wants may be different. When this happens, it can be very difficult for people with an intellectual disability to stand up for what they think is best for them.

Even when people move out of institutions they may carry with them the fear that they will some day go back into the institution. The chapters in this part of the book show that sometimes people do move in and out of institutions over their lives. The reasons for this are different for each person. So Tom Allen's age and health made it difficult for him to live in the community, while Rowan moved into and out of different kinds of institutions as his family continued to try and find him the place where he could live a happy and fulfilling life. He now lives in the community.

In the early 1990s I spent two years of field work exploring what the process of moving out from a large institution for people with intellectual disabilities meant to a group of women, their families and carers (Johnson 1998a; see also Chapter 3). This research involved close contact with the women themselves and with the team closing the institution. At the time I was somewhat surprised at the lack of information and research about the actual process of closing large institutions. There was a great deal of literature about the institutions themselves (Blatt 1981; Goffman 1961; Wolfensberger 1975) and a growing body of work on the lives of people who had left them (Barron 1989; Crossley and McDonald 1980; Potts and Fido 1991). In terms of institutional closure, much was written from a policy perspective (Collins 1992; Conroy and Bradley 1985; Dunt 1988; Knapp *et al.* 1992; Korman and Glennerster 1990) and some literature documented the legal struggles in which people had engaged in order to leave (Rothman and Rothman 1984). However, there was little that captured the attempts to make the *process* of moving out itself understandable.

At the institution in which I was based I watched as the closure team reconnected women in the institution with families from whom they had often been long separated, held consultations about their future lives and then managed the actual decision making which determined where they would live. The closure team had good intentions and had given much thought to designing ways of 'moving out' that would reflect the emphasis on rights that underlay institutional closure. In practice, however, lack of resources and time, and the pressure of management issues, cut across many of the well-laid plans (Johnson 1998b). As a result there was an absence of voices from the women who lived in the unit where I was based, and a gap between the conceptual design for closure, which called for ordered processes and rituals, and the messiness of its implementation.

Many of the issues I encountered in my experience of institutional closure are reflected in the chapters in Part II of this book. However, the authors of these chapters describe more diverse experiences of moving out than I was able to capture in my case study. In particular, they reflect differences in the time at which people left the institutions and the culture in which the 'moving out' occurred. In this chapter I draw out some key themes from these chapters and reflect on how these may provide guidance in future processes of institutional closure.

Fighting for the right to move out

The chapters in Part II reveal that for some people the process of moving out was an individual struggle. It did not come as part of government policy that closed the institution in which they lived. Rather, it was the result of an individual's expressed need. In Chapter 7 Tom Allen graphically describes the court case that led to his movement into the community. His appearance in court, even with support, was not easy. It occurred in opposition to the views of his brother who had been his main advocate. It meant that an old man who had spent most of his life in institutions had to confront the foreign rituals of court. And, more than that, he had to describe in detail the abuse and poor quality of life he had experienced in the institution. Reading his chapter, I was very aware of the courage this must have taken. When he went to court, Tom was still living in the institution which he so strongly criticized. What consequences might that have for him? Further, the difficulties Tom might have experienced in his court appearance should not be underestimated. For example, Amanda Tuttleby, an Australian woman with an intellectual disability who took legal action to obtain her rights as a Scout leader in Australia, has vividly described the confusion and anxiety she experienced in a court appearance and its subsequent effects on her life (Tuttleby with Johnson 2000).

Further, most of us can make choices about where we live and with whom. However, Tom had to justify his right to spend his last years living in the community to a legal forum. Essentially, the decision was not his to make but was almost framed in legal terms of 'innocent' (able to live in the community) or 'guilty' (not able to live in the community).

A similar struggle to move out is apparent in the story in Chapter 9 from Ingiborg Eide Geirsdóttir. While she did not have to appear in court to assert her rights, she did have to win her place in the community against opposition from staff at the institution. Her story reveals how the very capabilities of some people with intellectual disabilities, which would make life in the community relatively easy for them, could actually be obstacles to their departure from an institution. Ingiborg was a worker within the institution and her decision to leave was not supported by staff because they valued her contributions. This experience was not unique. Other people with intellectual disabilities have had similar ones and it is difficult to know how many people spent their lives in institutions not because of their disabilities but because of their abilities (see, for example, Lodge and van Brummeten 2002; Walmsley 2000).

It is not only people with intellectual disabilities who have struggled to move out. Ethel Temby's account in Chapter 10 of her son leaving an institution demonstrates not only the importance of family commitment to the decision but also the need for family members to move on in terms of their ideas about the need for institutionalization of people with intellectual disabilities. Further, Ethel's story reveals that the decision for Rowan to leave the institution meant that he re-entered his family and they then had to make adjustments to his needs.

Emotional support in moving out

It is difficult to imagine what the process of moving out may mean to individuals who have lived much of their lives in a total institution. Perhaps the closest we can come to it is in the experience of separation and divorce where relationships may be severed, homes lost and geographical location changed. Yet even here we have some control over the processes: when they occur and how. We also have choices about how our lives will be lived. For people with intellectual disabilities, moving out can mean severing contact with all of those with whom they have lived, the loss of a home and sometimes of work or purpose.

A whole new life is offered in the community, but as chapters in Part II indicate, the choices they have about this are often limited. The support that people with intellectual disabilities need to deal with the often unavoidable anxieties and stresses involved in moving out has not been well documented in the literature. Perhaps this is because those of us who have supported institutional closure have not appreciated that while total institutions may often have offered a poor quality of life to residents, they were often the person's whole life experience. Or perhaps it is because our views of people with intellectual disabilities still deny them the capacity to feel the grief and anxiety that the rest of us feel in similar situations. The accounts of moving out in Part II reveal yet again the lack of emotional support that is given to people by carers or service providers. None of the writers in this book show evidence that counselling or emotional support on a formal level was ever offered to them. A house, a group home or a room becomes available in the community and the person moves out of the institution and into a new life. Sometimes people are able to retain some contact with people they knew, at other times this is lost.

Only in the chapter by Ethel Temby is there a stress on the need to provide some structured way to make the transition easier. So for her son, contact with the institution where he had lived was maintained until he decided that he no longer wanted it.

Moving in and out and in and out...

As large institutions close there is a temptation to see the process of moving out as something that happens once in a person's life. Perhaps this is more likely to be so now than in the past. However, three chapters in Part II of this book demonstrate that moving out is not necessarily something that is a unique event in someone's life.

The reasons for this are different for each person. Tom had moved across several institutions during his lifetime. His stories in this book repeatedly describe how the process of moving out meant different things to him at different times. Sometimes he moved to seek a better quality of life in another institution, sometimes he moved because of a desire to live more freely in the community. For Tom, even when moving out was a fact of life, the thought of being moved back into the institution was a constant threat and fear. Whether or not people do move in and out of institutions in reality, they may internalize the fear of what this has meant to them in the past.

For Rowan, the process of moving in and out is a repeated theme throughout his mother's chapter. The driving force behind these moves was to find a place where Rowan could lead a fulfilling and happy life. Moving out of an institution into life with his family was one step. But the failure of the services to be able to provide him with an interesting life in the community led to him 'moving in', to an alternative, but still to some extent institutionalized, environment. Years later he again moved out. Rowan's experiences raise questions about the capacity and willingness of services in the community to provide continuing support for people as they inevitably go through different life stages.

Many of us experience a flow of jobs, relationships and accommodation over our lifetimes, but the process of moving in and out of institutions is quite a different experience. Sometimes, even when it is driven by good intentions, it may not be the desire of the person being moved, and the threat of moving into an institution can cast a shadow over the achievement of living a freer lifestyle in the community.

Family support

The women with whom I worked in the institution had diverse degrees of family support. Some saw family members on a regular basis but more than half had little or no contact with them. Family members' perceptions of their relative became extremely important when they were involved in decision-making about moving out. For some women, the process was made easier by the positive approach of family members. For others, family views about their future lives led to their being reinstitutionalized.

The chapters in Part II of this book reveal the importance yet again of positive support by family members for people with intellectual disabilities involved in the process of moving out. While Tom Allen's brother did not support his move into the community, he did not actively oppose it. Had he done so, or had Tom been less articulate or forceful, the result may have been very different. Ingiborg's family has been a support to her during the process and since her move into the community. Ethel Temby's chapter illustrates the struggle of a family to find a good life for and with Rowan, and the constancy of the support that they have offered him. Now in her eighties, Ethel has yet again been involved in the process of assisting Rowan to move out.

The part that families can play in facilitating the process of moving out is clear. However, it is also apparent that families can wield a great deal of power in relation to both the individual and the services that he or she uses. Perhaps the key issue here is the weight that is given by service providers to family power in decision-making around moving out. There is no doubt that in some instances family involvement is extremely important to the individual. However, it is also apparent from these chapters that families' needs or views are not always in agreement with those of the person with a disability. Family members may have other needs and agendas which run counter to either the rights or the best interests of the person. It is difficult in these situations to know how to manage the processes of moving out. Who should have decision-making power? What are the consequences for the individual of opposing family expectations and views? What supports should be given to families to help them to make decisions on behalf of or with their family member? None of these questions seem to have been answered satisfactorily in accounts of institutional closure.

The gap between concept and practice

Christine Bigby's chapter (Chapter 8) illustrates clearly the gaps that can exist between the concept of how moving out should happen and the obstacles encountered by those who implement it. Failure to provide contact between the people with disabilities and the people who will support them in new lives can have devastating effects on both the person and the morale of care givers. Bigby's chapter also reveals how the processes of individual instances of moving out are shaped and governed by policies and ideologies in the broader political context. For example, the move towards the provision of contractual arrangements between government and services can lead to a failure to take into account the individual needs and desires of people moving from institutional life to the community.

It is also apparent from Bigby's chapter that the process of moving out is complex and difficult for those who are responsible for it. Behind each individual who packs his or her bags to leave the institution is an army of people who have consulted, developed files, provided information, located houses and day services, tried to link people with new services and briefed new staff. Little of this complexity and planning is shared with the people who are subject to institutional closure. The accounts by the people with disabilities in this section reveal that for them the process of moving out had to do with an offer of a house or a flat. I am left wondering how different this experience is for them from the one where they were offered a 'bed' in an institution.

In the design of institutional closure there still seems little capacity to involve people directly in the planning of where, with whom and how they will live after they move into the community. Nor is there very much evidence from Christine Bigby's chapter of efforts to ensure that people meet with and have some choice about those who will be either living with them or caring for them in their new services.

The costs of moving out

All change involves some grief and letting go of past events and circumstances. For some of the people who have written of their experiences in this section of the book, the losses had to do with relationships. For Ingiborg, however, the loss was both intimate and invasive. Before she could move out of the institution she had to undergo sterilization. It is salutary to realize that this condition on moving into the community is not something in the far distant past but was experienced by a woman who is in her early 50s at the time of writing.

The communal fear that people with intellectual disabilities pose some form of genetic danger to the rest of the population if they should have children was reinforced by the eugenics theory early last century (Johnson and Tait 2003; Rose 1979). Its consequences included the institutionalization of many people with intellectual disabilities. The remnants of this now discredited theory and its associated fear can be found in the struggle that many people with intellectual disabilities still have to enjoy active sexual lives (Johnson *et al.* 2000; Walmsley and Johnson 2003). Ingiborg paid a high price for her flat in the community. I wondered what this imposed decision about sterilization really meant to her. She talks of not having children, but what effect did it have on her to be regarded as someone not capable of being a parent or, worse, someone whose fertility was regarded as a community danger? Her community actually told her that in order to live with others she must not have children. There are no other groups in the community that have been subjected to this kind of proscription. The process of moving out can bring into sharp relief the ways in which we still constitute the subjectivity of people with intellectual disabilities.

Conclusion

People who have moved out, move on. New lives. New relationships. Yet they carry with them the fears that are part of the process, fears about moving back in, fears about the impermanence of freedom. After all, social changes over which they had no power led to their institutionalization and then later to their deinstitutionalization. There is little certainty for them that the pendulum will not swing back. And for many of them the links to institutions are still there: in the struggle to make sense of community living, from which they were excluded; in work which may continue in an institutionalized setting or in the impermanence of the place in which they now live.

To move out, one must be inside, and that for many people with intellectual disabilities remains a possibility and a fear.

References

Barron, D. (1989) 'Locked away: Life in an institution.' In A. Brechin and J. Walmsley (eds) *Making Connections: Reflections on the Lives and Experiences of People with Learning Difficulties.* London: Hodder and Stoughton.

Blatt, B. (1981) *In and Out of Mental Retardation: Essays on Educability, Disability and Human Policy.* Baltimore, MD: University Park Press.

Collins, J. (1992) *When the Eagles Fly: A Report on the Resettlement of People with Learning Difficulties from Long Stay Hospitals.* London: Values into Action.

Conroy, J. and Bradley, V. (1985) *The Pennhurst Longitudinal Study: A Report of Five Years of Research and Analysis.* Philadelphia, MD: Temple University Developmental Disabilities Center.

Crossley, R. and McDonald, A. (1980) *Annie's Coming Out.* Melbourne: Penguin.

Dunt, D. (1988) *The St Nicholas Project: The Evaluation of a Deinstitutionalisation Project in Victoria.* Melbourne: Community Services Victoria.

Goffman, E. (1961) *Asylums: Essays on the Social Situation of Mental Patients and Other Inmates.* London: Peregrine Books.

Johnson, K. (1998a) *Deinstitutionalising Women: An Ethnographic Study of Institutional Closure.* Melbourne: Cambridge University Press.

Johnson, K. (1998b) 'Deinstitutionalisation: The management of rights.' *Disability and Society 13*, 3, 375–87.

Johnson, K., Hillier, L., Harrison, L. and Frawley, P. (2000) *People with Intellectual Disabilities: Living Safer Sexual Lives.* Melbourne: Australian Research Centre in Sex, Health and Society.

Johnson, K. and Tait, S. (2003) 'Throwing away the key: People with intellectual disabilities and involuntary detention.' In I. Freckelton and K. Diesfeld (eds) *Involuntary Detention and Civil Commitment: International Perspective.* London: Bloomsbury.

Knapp, M., Cambridge, P., Thomason, C., Beecham, J., Allen, C., Leedham, D. and Durton, R. (1992) *Care in the Community: Challenge and Demonstration.* Aldershot: Ashgate Publishing.

Korman, N. and Glennerster, H. (1990) *Hospital Closure: A Political and Economic Study.* Milton Keynes: Open University Press.

Lodge, C. and van Brummeten, F. (2002) *Kew Cottages: The World of Dolly Steiner.* Melbourne: Spectrum Publications.

Potts, M. and Fido, R. (1991) *A Fit Person to be Removed.* Plymouth: Northcote House.

Rose, N. (1979) 'The psychological complex: Mental measurement and social administration.' *Ideology and Consciousness 5*, 5–68.

Rothman D.J. and Rothman, S.M. (1984) *The Willowbrook Wars.* New York: Harper & Row.

Tuttleby, A. with Johnson, K. (2000) 'Thirty nine months under the Disability Discrimination Act.' In R. Traustadóttir and K. Johnson (eds) *Women with Intellectual Disabilities: Finding a Place in the World.* London: Jessica Kingsley Publishers.

Walmsley, J. (2000) 'Caring: A place in the world?' In R. Traustadóttir and K. Johnson (eds) *Women with Intellectual Disabilities: Finding a Place in the World.* London: Jessica Kingsley Publishers.

Walmsley, J. and Johnson, K. (2003) *Inclusive Research with People with Learning Disabilities: Past, Present and Futures.* London: Jessica Kingsley Publishers.

Wolfensberger, W. (1975) *The Origin and Nature of our Institutional Models.* Syracuse, NY: Human Policy Press (Syracuse University).

PART III

Living Outside

12

In the Community

Thomas F. Allen with Rannveig Traustadóttir
and Lisa Spina, USA

I moved into the community in March 1985 at the age of 72. I moved to an apartment with four other people with disabilities. I felt free and vowed never to live in an institution again. I have kept that promise. Two or three months after I moved out I got sick. I was in the hospital for seven days. It was my stomach. I think it was because I was afraid I would be sent back to the institution. I had nightmares about being back there. I think this fear upset my stomach.

My first year in the apartment was wonderful. I enjoyed very much being in a small home-like setting and living with a small group of people. I shared a room with John and we became good friends. It was a great disappointment when he moved to another group home and a young man moved in. We did not get along that well. We were too different. I also went on my first vacation to Florida for 11 days. It was such an adventure.

The staff in the apartment encourage us to speak up about what we want. I think that is good but it is difficult. In the institution I was punished when I spoke up and I kept thinking that my demands would lead to conflicts and punishments. I do not like conflicts and violence.

The apartment was better than the institution but my life was not all that much different in the community. Moving into the community did not bring me the freedom I had dreamed about. I was still isolated and could not do the things I wanted to do. The disappointment with my new life in the community is one of the greatest difficulties I have ever faced. I became desperate and depressed.

My friends became concerned and wanted to help me make my life better. They talked to the agency which came up with a very good solution. They hired a staff person to work with me Monday through Friday from nine o'clock in the morning till three o'clock in the afternoon. During this time I could do whatever I wanted with the help of my own staff person. Lisa was hired for the job. We became very good friends. She came into my life like an angel. She saved my life.

Tom Allen's story is continued from Chapter 7. Please see pp.34–35 and the Epilogue to Thomas F. Allen's Life Story on p.274 for a description of how the story was told and written.

Tom's story *continued*

On 9 March 1985 I arrived at my new home in a van from Syracuse Developmental Center (SDC). I had finally left the institution at the age of 72. I felt thrilled to see the van pull away without me! I felt free and vowed never to live in an institution again. I have kept that promise.

After I moved into the apartment many people from the agency came to see me. They wanted to know about my health and some other things. One person wanted to know what kind of recreational activities I wanted to do. I made a *big* list. I wanted to go to different places like to church; go shopping, out to eat, to plays and to ballgames; visit my family and explore downtown Syracuse. I looked forward to doing all these things. I was glad I could go to my church more often than when I was at SDC. Since I moved out, my friends from church pick me up just about every Sunday and take me back to the apartment. If my friends cannot take me, one of the staff at the apartment drives me to church. The apartment's van is especially made for wheelchairs so it is easy to get in and out of.

Fears and nightmares

Two or three months after I moved into the apartment I got sick. I had to go to the hospital for seven days. My stomach was acting up. I think it was because I was afraid this would not be a permanent arrangement. I was constantly afraid they would come and take me back to the institution. I feared they would change their minds and decide I could not live at the apartment. Sometimes I had nightmares about being taken back to SDC and I woke up in the middle of the night screaming: 'No, don't take me back!' I also had nightmares about being in the institution and being attacked by other inmates or being locked up or left to sit in a corner all day. I knew I would not survive if I went back to the institution. I knew I would die there and I did not want to die in the institution.

I think it was this fear that upset my stomach. What contributed to my fear was the fact that I was going back to SDC every day because the first two years I lived at the apartment I continued going to the workshop at SDC. Every morning, Monday through Friday, one of the staff members drove me over to the workshop where I had to work for six hours a day. I worked in a big room where I was assigned the job of counting and collating a certain number of papers into piles of 25 which someone else fastened together. I disliked having to go back to SDC every day. The work gave me something to do during the day but it was boring and meaningless. I wanted to do other things during the day than be at SDC. I enjoyed seeing some of my old friends who lived there and meeting some of the staff members but I did not want to work at SDC any longer.

In 1987, when I turned 75 years old, I was given an offer to retire. I decided I wanted to retire because I was tired and bored and I wanted to get away from the institution. There was a great retirement party for me. All my friends came. There were a lot of people there and I had a wonderful time. I think it is the best party I have ever been to.

My first vacation

My first year in the apartment was wonderful. I truly enjoyed being in a small home-like setting, eating at a family-scale table with a small group of people and living in a place that was like where 'normal' people live. About a year after I moved in I went on my very first vacation at 73. I flew to Florida for 11 days. It was such an adventure to be in an airplane. I went to Miami and stayed at my very first motel. I was amazed at what a real vacation was.

One of the best things about the apartment was that I felt safe there. I was getting elderly and was in constant fear for my safety in the institution. The other people who lived in the apartment were friendly and nice and I liked them. Especially John, my roommate, who became a good friend. It was a great disappointment to me when he moved to another group home. In his place a young man moved in. He used a wheelchair and worked in the community. We never got along that well. The age difference was too great and we had very different interests. It was hard to share a bedroom with someone so different from myself. I also found as I grew older that I had less tolerance for such things as loud rock music.

Speaking up is hard

The staff in the apartment encourage us to speak up about what we want and how we feel about things. I think that is good but it is difficult for me. When I was in the institution and they yelled at me, I listened to them but did not say anything back. If you said anything back you were in serious trouble and could be punished just for saying what you wanted. Now, when I'm encouraged to say what I want, it is hard for me. I do not like conflict. I am a man of peace. Conflicts and fights bother me very much. In the institution I learned that to keep the peace you had to keep quiet about your needs and wishes. If I made demands on my own behalf it usually led to conflicts and punishments. In the apartment I am encouraged to make demands on my own behalf and say all my wants and needs, but it is hard. I do not trust that it will be all right to speak up. I keep thinking it will result in conflict.

My sister Marion and my brother Neal came to visit me at the apartment after I moved in. Marion used to live in California but she has moved to a small town close to Canisteo, where we grew up. It was good to see her. I had not seen her in a long time. Both Neal and Marion liked the apartment and said they were glad to see me there. This was much better than the institution, they both said. Neal said he was glad I insisted on moving out. It was good to hear him say that.

Disappointments

After I moved into the apartment I did go out a little more than when I was in the institution. But not much more. The staff at SDC had been taking us out into the community quite often. In the apartment I went to a few more ballgames and a few more restaurants. But I was not going out as much as I wanted to because I kept spending all my days at SDC. After I retired from the workshop I hoped I would be going out more but that did not happen. Instead, I sat around in the apartment alone with one staff person most of the day and had little to do except watch TV or play music. The other residents were out working all day and most of the staff did not come to work until after the other residents came back from work. There were not enough staff to take me out during the day. The staff who were working during the day had other things they had to do.

As it turned out, my life was not much different in the community than it had been in the institution. I think that this disappointment with my new life in the community was one of the greatest difficulties I had ever faced.

Moving into the community did not bring me the freedom I had dreamed about. I was still quite isolated. All the lists I had made about all the things I wanted to do seemed to have disappeared. I did not have the possibility to visit my brother and sister or other members of my family as much as I had hoped. I really wanted to see one of my nephews in Kentucky who is a minister. He is Bob's son. The plane tickets were expensive and I saved for a long time to have enough money to go on a vacation. But when one of the staff went to the bank for me to get the money I had saved for the ticket to Florida, it was gone. Someone had taken it all. One of the staff probably. I was crushed that someone could do that. It turned out all right though because all my friends chipped in and came up with enough money for the ticket. It was a great disappointment that this happened. I would expect such things in the institution but not in the community.

Depression and despair

Moving out of the institution did not bring me the life I had hoped for. I became desperate and depressed. What was most difficult for me to face was that the apartment was in some ways not that different from the institution. Don't get me wrong: I would never move back to the institution and I am glad to be out. But there are still things at the apartment that are similar to the institution. For one thing, the apartment is not like my own home where I can decide things and do what I want. I can have my say and express my wishes but the staff make the rules for the most part and make the decisions. Another thing that also bothers me is that staff come and go all the time, just like in the institution. As soon as I have learned to like the staff, chances are that they will quit. Many of the staff are young people and sometimes they play loud music in the evening. Sometimes when there are young men and women working the same shift they are more occupied with each other than with assisting us who live here. Sometimes they chase each other around the apartment with a lot of noise and don't seem to care how we feel about all that noise and excitement. I like these people and enjoy seeing them happy but in my old age I want to have peace and quiet in the evening.

Losing hope

I was getting old and slow and I didn't have many teeth left so it took me a long time to eat. Some of the staff did not like helping me eat. They thought it took too long and I could feel they didn't want to be bothered. Therefore, I sometimes did not eat as much as I should and occasionally I didn't eat at all. When a staff member said: 'Do you want something to eat Thomas?' and I knew they didn't want to be bothered feeding me, I just said I didn't want any food. I knew it was not good for me because my stomach problems require that I eat regularly. But somehow I didn't care. I was getting very tired and disappointed. My health was failing. I was losing weight and, what was worse, I was losing hope. I did not even want to talk. I wanted to die.

The 'retirement programme'

My friends became concerned about me and started thinking about how my life could be improved. They talked to the agency and asked what could be done and the agency came up with a wonderful solution. They created a 'retirement programme' which meant I would have my own staff person who would only work with me Monday through Friday from nine in the morning to three in the afternoon. This person's task was to assist me in what I wanted to do during the day. This would mean that I would be able to get out more often, go places and do what I wanted to do every day.

This sounded almost too good to be true and I accepted the offer of this programme. Lisa, one of the resident counsellors, who had already been working in the apartment for about a year, applied for the job. Lisa became my 'retirement programme' in 1987 and we found out right away that we really got along very good together. My life changed for the better again. Lisa came into my life like an angel. She saved my life.

Tom Allen's story continues in Chapter 17 on p.205.

13

'I've Got My Freedom Now'

Memories of Transitions Into and Out of Institutions, 1932 to the Present Day

Victor Hall with Sheena Rolph, UK

My name is Victor Hall and I was born in a workhouse in Norfolk in 1932. I was then moved with my mother and my brother to a colony (later, hospital) for people with an intellectual disability because they said my mother was not well. My father was not well either, and in the end I never did meet him. My mother went to another hospital and she came to visit us on some Sundays. But then she went to live in Canada with her sister.

I stayed in the hospital for a long time and then they moved me into Blofield Hall, a hostel close by which was a halfway house. I had much more freedom there and so I liked it better. I had hobbies – taking photos, keeping budgies, and my own piece of garden – and we could go into Norwich (the nearest city) on the bus or train every fortnight to go to football matches. We went on holidays to the seaside and we went out to play sports in other places. I did lots of different jobs and I got paid for them. I worked back in the hospital on the wards, serving food and looking after the children and the clothes store. I also worked in the tailor's shop in Blofield Hall mending clothes. I liked most of these jobs – sometimes I was almost like staff! But there were some things I didn't like about the hostel: they used to lock the doors up at night times; we couldn't go to bed what time we liked; if one boy was naughty, we were all stopped from going into Norwich.

Then came the big change for me: I was moved out of Blofield Hall in 1972 to live in Norwich with my brother. The hospital social worker found me a job as a kitchen porter in a hotel and we lived in a chalet in the hotel gardens. At first it was strange. I took time to settle. But then it was all right. I felt I had my freedom then. And I felt I'd got my own job: I left the hotel and ended up with a council flat and a job in a fish-and-chip shop which I had for 20 years – I only retired two weeks ago! I have always had a busy life in Norwich – going to the social club, going on holidays with my friends and the club, going to conferences and going to Adult Education classes.

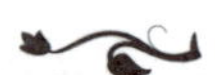

Sheena writes: I met Victor in 1997 when he agreed to help me with my research into the history of community care for people with intellectual disabilities in Norwich, Norfolk. I was particularly interested in his life, as his was a story of complicated multiple transitions on his journey to independence. I interviewed Victor on several occasions, and we also met regularly with a memories group to talk about the past and to look at Victor's many photographs, which are a unique documentation of a historical era. More recently, Victor and I met to talk specifically about this chapter, and in the course of that conversation he filled in many of the gaps in his story and brought it up to date. For this chapter I have adapted the interview format and changed it into a narrative, using Victor's own words as much as possible. Victor and I have read it through together and he added some things and took out others that were not right. He is now happy with his story. Sometimes we talk about places in the story that may not be known by the reader. When this happens I have put explanatory comments in brackets.

Victor's story

How I ended up in an institution

I was born in Gressenhall Workhouse in Norfolk in 1932. My mother was put in there but my father wasn't, although they were married – he is on my birth certificate. Then me and my brother Basil had to go into Little Plumstead [a colony for people who were in those days labelled 'mental defectives', later renamed as a hospital] because my mother had to go in there as she wasn't well. It was in the countryside. We went in there when we were very small, into the children's ward. My father wasn't well either but he had hoped to move near to us so that he could visit his sons whom he called in a letter his 'two bright boys'. But then they moved my mother to another hospital, and me and my brother stayed behind. In the end I never met my father. My mother visited us sometimes. I can remember her coming on some Sundays. Then she got discharged from the hospital and she left England to go and live with her sister in Canada. I can remember the day she came to say goodbye. We went to Great Yarmouth for the day – and we saw the bridge go up – I've got a photo of it. And that's the last time I saw my mother. She wrote to me sometimes, but she died in 1984.

Life in the hospital

The staff looked after me when I was little. We had a school on the ward in a small room with desks and a blackboard, and we had to copy things out on paper. The nurses taught us. I was on M2, then on M4. When I was older I worked in the mess room – the staff room – cleaning and washing up. Then they put me in the painters' workshop as a helper: I held the bottom of the ladders as they were dangerous.

A big change in my life: Moving out to Blofield Hall

Moving out of Little Plumstead Hospital and into Blofield Hall [a health authority hostel and halfway house for men, one mile from the hospital] was a very big change for me. It was a new kind of life. I remember my first days there. The staff took me up in a minibus and they showed me round the rooms. I was in a room with six boys and my brother. It was a grand large house with big gardens. I was pleased about moving there because we could go out – we had more freedom than in Plumstead.

HOBBIES AND SPORTS

I had a hobby there: I had budgies...yellow, green and blue. Me and my brother Basil went to the pet shop in Blofield village and bought them – one was called

Joey. We had to look after them and feed them twice a day. Basil taught me to take photographs, and I bought a camera. I have got about ten albums full of our photographs which show our lives in Blofield Hall.

Blofield Hall had lovely gardens – there were lots of daffodils on the main drive. Another hobby I had was that Basil and I used to do the garden. We had allotments – we used to have a piece of garden each. I used to dig it and we used to be able to garden by ourselves. Basil and I grew vegetables and then he went out selling them round the hospital. My own garden was one of the things I liked about Blofield Hall.

I liked watching football, and we were allowed to go into Norwich [seven miles from the hostel] once a fortnight and go to football matches. Sometimes I went on the bus, sometimes on the train. We had to ask the staff and put our names down before we could go out, but I liked it because I felt I had more freedom.

And at Blofield Hall I played sports organized by the hostel chaplain. I was on the snooker and darts teams and the outdoor bowls team. We went out to play bowls in Great Yarmouth and Ipswich, and we beat Ipswich! In 1972 I won a medal at bowls in Cambridge. We used to go out in a coach to play bowls – and I liked going out because we hadn't gone out before when we were in the hospital.

We had a social club in Blofield Hall, and me and Basil served behind the bar selling beers. I remember the party on 'open night' and dances and discos and sing-songs round the piano. The boys could bring their girlfriends from the hospital in for visitors' evenings.

We used to go on holiday from Blofield Hall: we went off in big coaches to camp at the seaside in Caister and Yarmouth, all the boys in big tents together for four weeks. For the first two weeks we had to look after the children – we went on the coach with them to parks, we went on the beach with them and we had to tidy them up. Then the second two weeks was without the children. I went on the beach and went swimming, and Basil and I went into the town to look around the shops. We went to the Great Yarmouth Public Baths once a week! Now I really miss those camping trips with all the boys.

JOBS IN BLOFIELD HALL

We had work to do in Blofield Hall. I had lots of different jobs. We had to clean the rooms first thing in the morning and clean the sinks. Then they asked me, 'Do you want a job in Plumstead?' and I said, 'Yes', and they put me on M7 [a ward in the hospital] then, and they gave me a job working in a dormitory making beds. And when they were short-staffed, then I looked after the patients. I worked in the kitchen on M7 too, serving out. We wore white coats and we served meals on wheels to the patients. We got paid in Blofield Hall on Fridays.

When they were short-staffed I used to work on the children's wards and took them for walks. I also kept the keys to the clothes cupboard. When parents came I had to get the children ready, and when nurses wanted clothes out of the cupboard, they had to ask me for the keys. I was like staff really! And I had to wear a white coat or jacket.

I enjoyed these jobs and I didn't get fed up. I got a lift to the hospital in the mornings but often had to walk back to Blofield Hall at night down a long road in the dark and that was scary!

As well as jobs in the hospital, I worked back at Blofield Hall in the tailor's shop. I found it quite difficult. We sewed on buttons, did mending, that sort of thing. I worked on the sewing machines, and it was before I had my glasses and it was a hard job threading the needle. They were peddling machines, the old-fashioned ones. I remember I worked on stitching pairs of trousers up. It was a long time ago. I also worked for a time in the carpenter's shop where someone showed me about planing wood.

Another job we had was going out to help a local farmer. He came down and said he wanted volunteers to help picking up potatoes on a Sunday. About six or seven of us went. We had pay packets, but we handed the money in to the staff and then any time we went out, we asked for some money. On a Friday we asked: 'Can we have some money to go down the city?'

THINGS I LIKED ABOUT BLOFIELD HALL

Living in Blofield Hall felt more like a young man's life. I liked going out, and into Norwich and other places. I liked my garden and my hobbies. I was pleased to move there because we were the 'high grades' and I liked being with the boys. My jobs were good, I earned a pay packet and I was like staff. I felt: 'I've got my freedom now.'

THINGS I DIDN'T LIKE ABOUT BLOFIELD HALL

There were also many things I didn't like about Blofield Hall. The worst one was, we were locked up night times. They locked the doors up at about eight o'clock or nine o'clock – the main entrance door. They turned the key. I didn't like that at all.

We couldn't go to bed what time we liked: we had to turn the television off at ten o'clock. We had to queue for the bathroom and had a bath only once a week. And we had to get a towel from the office for a bath – all rolled up. We got clean clothes handed out once a week after the bath. We didn't cook our own food – or choose it. We had stews and semolina, I remember, and it came over from the hospital in a hot trolley.

If one boy got wrong, we all got wrong: we were all stopped from going into Norwich on a Saturday. That spoilt it for the others. That wasn't fair. And another thing: when we used to go into Norwich we had to write our names down, that sort of thing. We had to be back before eight o'clock because we used to have roll call, and if we weren't back in time and our names weren't ticked off in time, we couldn't go to Norwich again. If a boy was naughty, the punishment was he was sent to bed early or his money was stopped.

I didn't feel it was my home. I wanted to get out. Because they locked the doors up at Blofield Hall.

THE FINAL MOVE: IT FELT A BIT STRANGE

In the early 1970s they found me a part-time job cleaning floors in The Clover Leaf Café in Norwich. So I went in on the bus every day from Blofield Hall. This was to help me to get ready to move out completely. In 1972 came the big change: I moved out of Blofield Hall.

The hospital social worker got me a full-time job in the Eiger Hotel with Basil, and she took me in the car to the Eiger. I was a kitchen porter and I had to clean the pans up – and wash plates and saucers. It was hard work. Usually I worked from 10am to 3pm and also worked night times. Sometimes if it was a wedding we stayed washing up till 2am! We had one day off a week.

Basil and I lived outside of the hotel in a chalet in the garden. It was cold at first as it didn't have any heating. There were no radiators, so then they put in some with thermostats. It was nice, though, as we had two bedrooms, one each, a sitting room and a bathroom, and we bought a black-and-white TV. We went out down the shops for the papers in the morning; we went out to the city when we liked. A bit different from living with all the boys in Blofield Hall!

It all felt a bit strange at first. It took a long while for me to settle. In a piece I wrote for a magazine in 1986, I said that doing just what I liked at first seemed strange and I missed friends, missed looking after people and looking after the children (Hall 1986). But then it was all right. I had a month's trial at the hotel and then they discharged me from Blofield Hall. I didn't know what it would be like to live outside Blofield Hall after so many years. The new life was very strange – but I liked it a lot: nobody locked up at night.

The new life

There were more changes and I had some difficulties. I had to leave the Eiger Hotel when the management changed. So I went down the job centre and got myself a job at Sprowston Hall Hotel, again as a kitchen porter. My social worker helped me into lodgings until the council found me a flat in 1980. The job was hard, though: I had to walk back home every night at about 2am, although sometimes they would give me a lift back in a taxi. But it was long hours, so I left and went on the dole.

I had made some friends – some girls in lodgings near me. One of them found me a job in a fish-and-chip shop – Joe's Fish Shop. I felt I'd got my own job then. I got the chips ready and I cleaned the chip shop floor. The fish shop was the best job out of all the others. I worked hard and I got paid. I worked there for 20 years and I retired at the age of 71. I sometimes don't get up until 9.30 in the morning now!

I'm still in the same flat. My brother came to live with me there until he died. I have a small garden and I have nice neighbours and friends nearby. We have parties and this summer we went on holiday together to the seaside. Three of us went – one can't walk as he is in a wheelchair, so we had turns in pushing him. People talk to me and I help my neighbours if they are ill.

How I feel about life on the outside

In my article I wrote: 'People treat me like a man now, not like a boy. Nobody tells me "Do this! Do that!" Nobody tells me what time to come in' (Hall 1986). At first when I came out I was helped by a social worker, but I don't have a social worker now.

I still have some old friends from Blofield Hall and I made new friends too. I joined a social club – the Wednesday Club that's now called 'Build' – and I was voted on the committee for a few years. I liked that. I go every week and now they have made me a volunteer with a volunteer's badge. I go every week to the Thursday Club – 'Steps' – where we sit round in a circle and talk about things. I go with Build to conferences at the Open University. I like going to Adult Education because I never learned to read or write in the hospital. In Adult Education I've done 'Word Power' and now I'm on 'Dictionary Practice'.

My only difficulty being out has been my speech. Some people don't always get what I am saying. But when they get to know me they do. My glasses help me now and I'm learning new words.

I've seen a lot of changes in my life and now Plumstead Hospital is closed and Blofield Hall is empty. It is going to be turned into flats and houses. That long dark road is still there, though! But it's all overgrown now. I like my freedom: I just go out, up the road, catch a bus, go to Adult Education. I like my flat – I've got a back garden where I grow things.

Moving out was the biggest change for me. What I say is that I'd rather be out than in; being out is much better – even though it was strange at first.

Conclusion

Sheena writes: Victor's life story gives us a glimpse into both the local and national history of intellectual disability in England, and the effects upon him of changing times, attitudes and policies. His incarceration in institutions in the first place was the result of the certification of his mother under the 1913 Mental Deficiency Act, which enacted legislation to segregate people 'ascertained' as having an intellectual disability in large institutions or to place them under close surveillance in the community. The infantilizing language of the 1960s is echoed in Victor's description of his friends in the hostel as 'boys'. His many different jobs, though he appreciated and enjoyed them, could be seen as exploitation of on-hand cheap labour in the hospitals, without which they could not run economically. The isolation of the hospital and the segregation of the sexes harked back to the eugenicist policies of 1913. Changing national policy was stated in the 1971 White Paper which declared renewed support for care in the community as opposed to institutional care. The new policies were echoed in the transition for Victor in 1972 from Blofield Hall, the halfway house, to independent living in the hotel chalet in Norwich. Most dramatically of all, today much of Little Plumstead Hospital, including the wards he mentions – M7, M4 and M2 – is now overgrown with weeds and grasses, about to be bulldozed in favour of a new housing estate. Blofield Hall still stands – but is boarded up in anticipation of another role as flats and maisonettes.

The symbols of Victor's freedom, however, still remain: Joe's Fish Shop on Magpie Road, and his council flat, full of *half* a lifetime's possessions. We can hope, therefore, that times have changed and that somebody like Victor would not be institutionalized today, simply because his mother was poor, working class and experiencing difficulties as a parent. She and his father would be helped to bring up their 'two bright boys' together. A false hope? Victor's story, and many like it, can perhaps stand as a reminder of the past and a warning that great vigilance is needed if we are not to return to it.

Reference

Hall, V. (1986) 'Moving out.' *CMH Newsletter 47*, Winter, 4.

14

'Gone Fishin''

From Institutional Outing to Real Life

Emil Johansen with Kristjana Kristiansen, Norway

The authors have chosen not to have a plain English summary of this chapter.

Kristjana writes: Emil is a fisherman who lives in a small village in northern Norway. Emil has an intellectual disability and some physical impairments, and he spent much of his early life in an institution. This chapter tells some of his life story. Emil and Kristjana have spent many hours visiting each other informally, having conversations and going fishing. Emil did most of the talking, and Kristjana wrote notes and used a tape-recorder. In order to make this into a life story, they agreed to reorganize things Emil had said into sections, according to historical sequence. The introductory headings for each section are paraphrased questions from Kristjana. They have been reformulated using Emil's voice in the 'I' form and Kristjana's in the 'you' form, as an attempt to preserve the position of Emil as storyteller. The content, however, is wholly Emil's own words, but with considerable reduction. Emil helped select what he thought was most relevant and he approved the final version in Norwegian, which was then translated into English by Kristjana. Emil decided not to use his real name in this story. He discussed it with his sister and they thought their mother would be unhappy about it if she saw the story in a book. Instead, they decided to use the names of two of their friends, Emil and Gertrud. All other names of people and places have also been changed.

Emil's story

You asked about my life today...what's good and not so good. You want me to tell you what I do now.

Life is much better than before. So first, I'll tell you some things I remember about my life before. I don't remember me, when I was a little boy. Except some things. I remember my sister. I remember the building I lived in. My sister was also at Himmelfjell [an institution]. She was always nice to me and visited me. I have trouble with my feet, couldn't walk. So we weren't in the same building. I was in a building with people who couldn't walk. Some were in bed all day. Mostly we just sat in chairs or on floor mats. Some people were quite sick, I think. They called our building the 'back building'. Sometimes it was hot. Sometimes at night it was cold. I don't remember being sad. Well, just sometimes. But maybe I was bored. It was difficult to sleep. Lots of people were noisy, and lights were on. Lights and noise, all the time. Later, in a dark room, I was scared. Now I like it. I like to sleep with the window open now.

My sister was always very pretty, always very clever. Her name is Gertrud. She worked in the laundry and sometimes in the kitchen. One of the staff in the kitchen liked her and he gave her chocolate. Then she gave it to me. I loved chocolate! I had never had it before. She told me this man liked her. And he 'played with her', she said. I guess she liked him. Later she told me he did things that weren't right. But then she was happy, always laughing and smiling. Everyone liked her. My sister and the chocolate were the best things from when I was there.

She talked to me all the time. And she understood me when I tried to talk. I asked her: 'Why can some people walk, some people not walk? Why don't people understand me when I talk?' My sister said: 'God just makes us that way.' Then she would laugh. She laughed about everything. She's always so happy. I often wished that my feet could walk. Some people in my building had very twisted feet. I was afraid my feet would get like that. I didn't have shoes. Sometimes in the winter, when I was older, I got to wear rubber boots. They weren't my boots. I thought my feet looked better.

My sister has a lovely smile and nice teeth. My teeth are bad. I had medicine before. I had seizures. That made my teeth bad. This is also why I have trouble talking. My sister believes in God. She said I should believe in God. She said she loves God. I asked her: 'Isn't he the one who gave me bad feet?' Sometimes I was in bed at night, hoping my feet would get better in the morning. I remember that.

When I got older I got pushed in a wheelchair to OT [occupational therapy]. I liked that. There were more people who could talk. We made things. We sang songs. I like singing. But I can't read. We went on outings. In a big bus. Sometimes

I couldn't go with them because I needed a wheelchair. Sometimes there weren't enough wheelchairs. But I went on most outings because I never went away on weekends or holidays like the others. They told me that. I liked the bus trips. Otherwise, I was always at Himmelfjell. The best outing was going fishing. I loved fishing! Every time they had an outing I asked: 'Can we go fishing?' They said: 'We already went fishing.'

I had a girlfriend at Himmelfjell. I met her at the OT building. Her name was Anna-Berit. She didn't talk much. She giggled a lot. I think I really loved her! I went to sleep thinking about her, you know! I used to dream about kissing her. She smelled so good. We could hold hands at OT. But no kissing! She would make things in OT and give them to me. I gave them to my sister, to take care of them. I never saw my sister's building, where she lived, but she said it was nicer. I never went in there. One time at the Christmas party, I kissed Anna-Berit. I got very excited, you know. We were outside. It was snowing. I was afraid someone would find us. Some staff saw us and were laughing. Then Anna-Berit went to Trondheim for Christmas to visit her mother. I missed her. It is the first time I cried, I think. I didn't think she'd come back. Anna-Berit was the first person I loved, I think. Except my sister.

I asked my sister many times about our mother. I asked: 'Didn't we have a mamma?' I went to sleep wondering why she didn't come to get us out. Other people went to visit their mother or families, or somewhere. Gertrud said our mother couldn't take care of us. And she had never visited us. Gertrud is older. She was seven years old when we went away from home. She thought we had another brother, maybe two brothers, maybe a sister. But she asked her boyfriend who worked in the kitchen. He told her about me, that I lived in another building. She didn't know that before. He said, no, we had no other brothers, no sisters. But Gertrud remembered someone else, another baby, when they first took us away. She said our mamma cried and wouldn't hug us goodbye. Someone drove us in a nice car, but Gertrud doesn't remember them. She said she forgot about me for a few years. She didn't know where I was. She was happy when she found me. Me too!

Later, I moved to a better building. They closed the back building. They tore it down. My new building was nicer. I got a new bed and a place to keep things. I had my own room, with five other guys next door. One guy I didn't like at all. He was always bothering me, running back and forth, and talking all night. My sister saved some things Anna-Berit had made for me. But I didn't want them. I wanted a radio. She said she heard we had some money and could get some things. I had listened to the radio before at OT. So I wanted a radio. I like music. When I was 33 years old, I got a radio for my birthday. My sister told the staff I wanted it. She said they used my money. I didn't know I had money.

You want to know about moving out?

When people started moving out, I got scared. I thought people moved out if their mother wanted them back. I didn't know where people went when they moved out. They just went away. Some people came back, like to visit. Anna-Berit moved out. She visited me. She came to OT, found me sitting at my same place. I was glad she came. She told everybody she was happy. Got a house, a garden. But then we didn't really like each other any more. I mean, she wasn't my girlfriend, really, after she moved out. I tried to ask her about being out but she didn't say much.

Then Gertrud moved out. She talked a long time about moving and she visited many places. She moved out long before me. After that I didn't like being at Himmelfjell. She visited me often. I once went to her new house but then she moved again. I kept asking when I could leave. 'Everybody's moving out', they always said. Well, I moved out. It happened very fast. They came one day, told me I was moving. Did I want to see the house? I asked, 'Where is it?' and 'Will I live with my mother?' I remember someone asked: 'Do you have a mother?' I thought, everyone has a mother, somewhere. They asked if I knew where she was. I said no. 'Who would I live with?' I asked. Gertrud visited me and she told me nothing about where I was going. Before, she told me everything. She knew things before I did. But when she came back and visited, she knew nothing about me. I always asked her: 'Can I live with you?' She said she didn't know if they thought that was okay. But we could maybe live nearby. I asked if she'd live with her sweetheart, the man with the chocolate. But she said he was gone. And he was a bad man and not her boyfriend any more. I don't know him. Then she got a new boyfriend.

They drove me to Norddalen. Me and my things. In 1994. I got my own house, by the river, near the church. Been here ever since.

My life now?

My life's okay now. First thing, I love fishing! Once, at Himmelfjell, we went on a fishing trip. I got no fish but I loved that trip! We had outings every week. Most people didn't like the fishing trip. The week after, I wanted to go fishing again. They said last week fishing, this week we visit a farm. I didn't want to see a farm. Every week I asked when we could go on a fishing trip again and they laughed. I got angry, sort of. I thought about fishing all the time. But now, I fish!

I have a girlfriend. She lives in Trondheim. Her name is Maria. She's very nice. I'm very lucky she wants me. We visit on weekends. Sometimes I take the train but usually she travels up here. I need help on the train. And sometimes my helpers don't want to go to Trondheim. It's far away. Maybe we'll live together, maybe next summer. She has a job in a shop. She wants to have a baby. But maybe I'm too old. I'm 42. She's only 29. She doesn't care, she loves me anyway! Her mother likes me. But she doesn't think we should get a baby. Maria has three cats. I would like a dog. But it's hard work to have a dog, I think. I don't really like cats.

I like to sing, too. I'm not very good but I try! I have lots of CDs. I know about karaoke. The words are written on the wall. I can't read but I know a lot of the words. Anyway, it's the others who really sing, not really me, you know? There's a place in Trondheim where we go to karaoke. Maria knows some other people who go there. So that's always a fun time.

I have lots of books, about fish. Of course! And also some videos, some from television programmes, about fishing. My dream is to fish in the winter. Out on the lake, on the ice. Have you seen it? The fish live under the ice. They live there all winter because there is water under the ice. The fishermen make a hole in the ice. And sit inside little huts. But my legs get too cold. My feet freeze. So in winter I watch fish videos. And Maria and I make popcorn and eat pizza. Sometimes we have some beer! We have lots of cosy evenings! If I had more money, I'd get some special fishing boots.

Fly-tying, do you know about that? I went to a course, to try to learn it. Much too difficult. A man, Sigurd, I met fishing by the river, he told me about the course. He drove me there. He was one of the instructors. But my hands don't work well enough to do it. You know, my fingers are twisted and don't go where I want. But it's fun to watch. I sit next to Sigurd. I went to his house for dinner. We ate fish. Of course! He showed me his fishing equipment. He makes good flies. He has a little room in his house, just to make flies, with lots of feathers and tools and things. Very difficult; some kinds of flies for spring, others for summer. It's because the fish know what kind of real flies there are. So we have to fool them, that's what Sigurd says. He doesn't talk much. But I think he is my best friend. I have maybe a hundred flies! Sigurd made many of them. I get them for Christmas, my birthday, when I have some extra money. We don't go fishing together often because he goes high up in the mountains. He has a mountain cabin there but I can't get up the path. But sometimes we go to another place where he has a little boat. He built a thing on the side of the boat to hold my fishing-rod. His wife is very nice. Her name is Torunn. But she doesn't like to go fishing. I sit with them in church on Sunday. They have a nice dog, named Topo. He's a retriever, that means he fetches things. He's a dog that goes bird-hunting with Sigurd. I don't think I want to go bird-hunting. Sigurd does that in October. He has other friends that go bird-hunting with him, at his mountain cabin. Torunn is there and makes food and knits. I saw photographs. Torunn knitted a big sweater for me, very warm. Maria wants to knit but she isn't so clever yet.

I go to church. It's next door to my house. I didn't go to church before I moved here. I can get there all by myself. Unless there's lots of snow and ice. I go Sundays, Easter, and times like that. Christmas is best, because we sing and there are beautiful lights. Saturday mornings, sometimes I help to clean the church classroom. Because Sigurd works there a little bit and he lets me help. And Torunn teaches children who come for a group. I help them with their snacks. We listen to stories about the Bible and she tells us what it means, and we talk about it. Maria doesn't like church. Sometimes Gertrud drops in. She shops at shops in my village on Saturday sometimes. Then we eat lunch together. She got married and lives in Kaldstad, not far away. She has a son. Sometimes I visit them but not very often. The train doesn't go there. She calls me every Sunday afternoon on the telephone. She loves to talk! Her son's name is Atle. He makes a lot of noise. I don't think he likes me but he's little. I wish he liked me. Gertrud says he'll like me when he gets bigger. Her husband's name is Harald. He works in the forests. They make paper out of trees. He has a good job. They have a little car, so it's difficult for them to drive me places. I wish I could visit them more often.

I like to live alone. I get some help with most things. Like shopping, cleaning, making food; and I need help to go out. Someone comes in the morning. And most afternoons and when I go out. It's different people all the time, but one guy named Jan-Eirik I like okay. But he doesn't like to fish. I'd like to go fishing more often. I live on the first floor. I know the two guys who live on the second floor. But we're not friends. My helpers also help them. Someone stays overnight there to help them. I can call them if I need help.

In the spring I sit on the veranda and watch the river. Sometimes I've seen the fish, the salmon, jump. Have you seen that? They jump in the air! Almost like flying! I have a video that shows it. Sigurd says they climb up the river. You have to be very clever to catch a salmon. Sigurd has got a few, one really big one. He has a photograph holding it. A huge fish! I got a big trout once. Mostly I get trout. I need help to fix the line. I have a thing on my wheelchair to help me hold the fishing-rod. And I need help when I catch a fish! Once I went fishing in a boat at sea but I got sort of sick. Bad waves! I like rivers and lakes best. I have a sign on my door, it's from England: 'Gone fishin'.' That's me, I'm a fisherman!

15

'Lady of the Well'

Memories of Vicki

Jen Devers, Australia

Vicki was my sister. I loved her very much. We grew up together in a country town in Victoria, Australia, with our parents and our four brothers and sisters. Although we didn't have much money, I remember lots of good times when we were both little girls. We played games in the shed where I was teacher and Vicki was my student, and we often dressed in the same clothes. When Vicki was 17 our mother became very ill and died. Vicki went to live in a large institution for people with intellectual disabilities. I feel very sad about the years she spent there.

After a long time the institution was closed and we were able to organize for Vicki to come and live near us. I was so excited at this change for all of us. I felt I would get to know my sister again. And I did. Vicki had some very good times in her house in the community. But there were also lots of problems. Neighbours didn't want to live near people with intellectual disabilities, Vicki became ill and was admitted to a psychiatric hospital and sometimes she had to go to day placements when she didn't want to because of lack of staff in the house. She also still had lots of medication, which really worried me. Her death was very sad. After dinner one night she choked on some meat which she was trying to eat. The staff tried to revive her but she died some days later. Although the coroner tried to find out why this happened to Vicki, I was left feeling that no one except her family really cared about her.

Vicki's story

> Vicki's family, the unit staff and the CCOR[1] convenor were all positive about her movement from Hilltop into the community. (Johnson 1998, p.33)

This closing sentence, in a book which documented the closure of the institution where Vicki had lived, understates the enormity of the second life-changing move for Vicki. Those words echoed the hopes and dreams that I had, as Vicki's sister and advocate, for her return 'home'. Hopes for the chance that I could ensure Vicki had the opportunities, choices and chances that she had been legally denied while surviving her 22 years in Hilltop. My dreams were that we would once more be linked as closely as we had been as children. Memories wash over me as I see us being dressed as twins, tottering up the shop on Christmas morning in our plastic Cinderella high-heeled shoes. Playing school in the woodshed, sharing kitchen duties. Just two sisters having fun. We also had moments of shared terror when fingers were stuck in jam tins or we nearly choked on the cricket-ball lollies that were around in the 1950s. As we got older the fun seemed to give way to pain of ridicule from the wider community, brought about by their ignorance of disability. We shared everything, even the pain.

In order to give a vignette of life for Vicki before she entered Hilltop, I will reflect back. Vicki was the fourth child in a family of eight. Like a lot of other families, money was in short supply, so we were seen as that poor family with the strange kid. Vicki was two years younger than me, although my mother created her own set of perceived twins by dressing us alike. My relationship with Vicki was a mixture of sister, carer, teacher and unofficial advocate. Many hours were spent playing school in the woodshed. Vicki would sit on a wooden fruit box while I tapped out 'cat', 'mat', etc. that had been chalked on the woodshed wall. She was a wonderful student.

Vicki's attendance at the local primary school seemed to be conditional on another member of the family being at school with her. Her school days were a mixture: acceptance, particularly from the girls who would like to mother her; ridicule from children who did not understand her.

We shared so much together: rooms, toys, baths and jobs at home. As awareness grew of just how difficult life was going to be, I even tried to shield her from the cruel taunts and teasing from other children. When Vicki turned 17, our mother's health had deteriorated to such a degree that her death was imminent. Having two younger siblings needing care, the doctor and Vicki's parents made the heartbreaking decision to move her to Hilltop. In the late 1960s there were virtually no services in the community to enable family members to stay within their homes and communities.

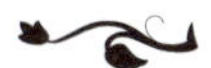

Vicki's passage leaving Hilltop was not as joyous an occasion as I envisaged. The unit in which she was being 'held' was indicative of the situation. Many women thrown together amid the emotional turmoil of uncertainty that was pervasive with the closure of a large institution for people with intellectual disabilities. The pain, anger and confusion within the unit were evidenced by the black eyes, scratches and bruising that Vicki bore on her face when we arrived to bring her home. The fact that she was constantly being badgered to wear shoes, when she clearly indicated that she did not want to, resulted in Vicki being very upset and unsettled before commencing the two-hour trip to her new home, close to us.

The home was a purpose-built five-bedroom house that Vicki shared with three male residents from Hilltop and another female from the local area. It appeared that no expense was spared in making this house a very comfortable, attractive and safe alternative accommodation to Hilltop. However, it was a little unsettling to discover that people in the neighbourhood had voiced their objections at having such a residence in the street. I hoped in time that their fears would be allayed once they got to know their neighbours. Unfortunately, this was not to be, as the Department of Human Services (DHS), in an effort to quell complaints from neighbours, had a block-out fence erected across the front of the house, obliterating any chance of neighbourly interaction. Once again, the people with intellectual disabilities were shut out of the community. A letter to the Human

Rights/Equal Opportunity Commission led to the fence being altered. It was not achieved without a good deal of stress, and in some sense set the scene for many a confrontation between some staff at DHS and myself.

Life for Vicki became a series of meetings, interviews and assessments. Words such as 'core costs', 'unit funding', 'high needs costs' all merged together to drive the direction of care that Vicki was to receive. Vicki was assessed as a person requiring high levels of care and therefore was placed in the high-cost category. The funding did not allow for residential staff to be paid for staying overnight on duty, which caused many difficulties when Vicki would wander around the house at night. The residential staff put in many unpaid hours during the times that Vicki found it difficult to sleep or was unsettled with pain. There was a constant battle about funding and how it was given. One example was day placement. A new day service was developed to provide meaningful daytime activities, which we hoped Vicki would attend. However, as a member of the steering committee, I found that the meetings seemed to be focused on arguing about funding and the lack of dollars to run the service in a way that truly reflected the needs of the clients.

After an initial settling-in period, Vicki became part of the access programme. This programme came about after two departmental employees pushed for funding to allow people returning to the community to have one-to-one support to look for and find enjoyable, preference-based activities. While this programme had enormous merit, it did have some drawbacks for Vicki. Visiting shopping plazas, noisy eateries and other areas where there were large numbers of people would often be overwhelming for her, and she would communicate her distress. I imagined how I would feel after living in a locked unit in an institution for 22 years and then confronting the noise, bustle and pace. Vicki was really struggling to adapt to the changes in her life.

I think sadly how frightening and lonely Hilltop must have been when Vicki went there after leaving the home environment that she knew so well.

When the access programme ended, pressure was exerted for Vicki to spend more time attending day placement. I did not feel that she was ready for the routine of being 'up and out' of home by a specific time each day. Naturally she did not respond meekly to instructions to be out of bed, showered, breakfasted and out the door by 8.45. Many times the taxi would be waiting in the driveway. It was such a sudden contrast from the long, lonely, timeless days spent wandering around Hilltop.

One thing Vicki never took to easily was change. This was not surprising given that many of the changes in her life had not been pleasant.

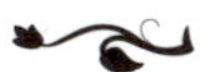

Space does not permit me to go into detail about all the experiences that Vicki had in the next eight years. Life in the community certainly offered her more opportunity to be involved in a wide variety of activities. Some she took to with great delight and she obviously enjoyed. She undertook others quite reluctantly. Long walks became an integral part of her day placement programme. After many years of pacing the locked unit at Hilltop, walking was not a habit that Vicki was able to stop even though she was living in a smaller confined area. This habit was to cause the residential staff great consternation.

At times her feet would become quite swollen and bruised, and she would not be able to rest her body. Sometimes she was ill, leading us to feel worried and concerned as we struggled to find the correct treatment. This in itself was to become a major issue between myself and staff from the department. I would not like to count the number of enemies that I made over the medication administered to Vicki. It appeared that the first action when she showed any behaviour change was to alter her medication. This was most unacceptable as records from Hilltop revealed that medications that had a sedating effect were widely and liberally administered throughout her many years in residence. I believed Vicki had a better chance of embracing her new life and relearning lost skills if she had a clear head. Many arguments and tears were shed over this issue. However, if I did nothing else I hope that I minimized the amount that she was prescribed.

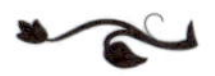

In the early days of Vicki's return, the new accommodation provided her with the security from physical abuse that Hilltop had failed to do. Vicki started to relax and enjoy her new living arrangements. There were many laughs to be shared at this time. There were many insights and discoveries for me watching the older Vicki deal with the newness of her life. As time went on, the newness gave way to the sameness and routine that seems to be the downside of living in a smaller institution.

On the face of it, this is what the residential unit drifted to. Staff started to come and go, and each one would bring and take something with them. Vicki had some wonderful relationships with some of the staff, although she was quite selective about those with whom she shared special times. Some of the staff developed a great affection for Vicki and she returned this by staying close, giving hugs and even making a cake for her favourite staff member. This staff member had given Vicki a most endearing nickname that Vicki would respond to.

Vicki had been having difficulty with sleeping for quite a while, and would get up and pace the house in the night, often disturbing the other residents. I would feel very anxious when these occasions arose, as I was aware of the other residents' rights to a full night's sleep.

Then her health started to fluctuate. Months would go by without any periods of difficulty for Vicki. Then would come the times when she would be so distressed and unsettled that we were puzzled as to how to ease her pain. A trip to the doctor's usually meant a new cocktail of drugs being prescribed for her. I often vehemently opposed this measure.

After returning from holidays, I was informed that Vicki had been admitted to the psychiatric unit of the hospital. My mind was racing in all directions: 'What was wrong with her? How was she feeling? Why had she been sent to the psychiatric unit?' I found out that Vicki had been screaming all day and night, and in order to reduce an explosive situation within the house she was removed. Staff argued that for her to receive appropriate services she had to be labelled with a psychiatric disability.

This admission started a pattern of Vicki's life that would continue until her death. The experience of her time spent in the psychiatric unit of the local hospital would create enough issues and material for a chapter in itself. They were heartbreaking times. I saw her being administered such large amounts of medication that she should have been unconscious for a month. Many times when we were out of view of staff I would just hold her and cry. Vicki would look at me and try to focus with her eyes, as if to say: 'What's happening? Why am I locked up in here?' The staff did not like or tolerate her. As her advocate, I often felt as if I were seen as a pest who got in their way and stopped them treating Vicki how they liked.

How it hurt when I noticed a huge bruise on Vicki's inner thigh when she was out of the psychiatric unit on a day visit with me. On investigation it emerged that a fellow patient had kicked her. I was furious to discover that the incident was not recorded and that no action had been taken: another reinforcement of my feeling that it didn't matter how she was treated. Alas, she could not speak up for herself. How vulnerable she was.

The psychiatric hospital had been closed three years earlier and a psychiatric unit opened within the newly built private (at that time) hospital and people were living in supported accommodation. It was no secret that if the hospital had still been operating, Vicki would have been admitted quick smart. It saddens me to acknowledge that would have been the only solution for those who cared for her. The thought that Vicki would have to endure being reinstitutionalized made me sick with worry. How could this happen, when she was taking time to adjust to living in the community? After 22 years of the same routine and setting at Hilltop, change would only come about gradually. It was quite evident that the staff in the psychiatric unit clearly saw it as not their role to have to nurse a person with an intellectual disability. Throughout Vicki's visits, sometimes for weeks at a time, in general hospital and the psychiatric unit, it became glaringly obvious that there was a lack of training for general nursing staff about the needs of people with intellectual disabilities. Attitudes ranged from fear to revulsion. After all, it is a reality of life that people with intellectual disabilities do at times need to be hospitalized and, therefore, nursed with the respect and care afforded to any other patient.

The days when Vicki was not well increased and she was not attending day placement as frequently, although there were times when the services argued about who was going to have her for the day. It was well known that the opportunity for people to stay at home for the day was not an option because of the staff rostering arrangements.

There were days that Vicki should not have been forced out to placement, but she was. This succeeded only in focusing negative attention on her. A book of bad behaviour exhibited by Vicki was being compiled. This system was used as a rationale to remove her from the house in the community where she still lived. A whole book could be written on the underhanded means and techniques that were used to manipulate Vicki's life. I discovered that to act as an advocate one has to be prepared for daily battles regarding medication, service delivery, accommodation, activities and, believe it or not, meals. For example, Milo [a chocolate-drink powder] was removed from the house as the residents were eating it. A directive was issued from the department that no more Milo was to be bought, even though the residents were paying the grocery bill. I dealt with that one by buying the largest tin of Milo I could find and gave that instead of Easter eggs. It left me wondering if any other options had been tried before totally banning Milo from the house.

The pressure of the clashes was unrelenting and at times I was stronger than others, but my focus always was Vicki's quality of life. At times it felt as though I was opposing every directive coming from the department, and with every good reason, as the changes and moves were always for the benefit of the department and hinged on dollars being spent. Control was always in the hands of the department. Staff members, employed at Vicki's home, were often frustrated by the limitations imposed by their employer. The limitations impacted on opportunities to create a fuller life for the people they were assisting. Over a period of time I watched some staff lose their enthusiasm for the role that they had undertaken, and the house slipped into a daily routine where boredom went unchallenged. The arrival of a new staff person provided an exciting diversion for a short time. I can still feel the poignant sense of hopelessness when I observed that Vicki's movements became robotic and were always directed by another person. Commands such as 'stop', 'turn' and 'sit' served to rob Vicki of her self-determination and her control over even minor actions.

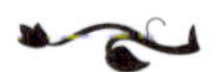

An emerging concern for me was the issue of ageing. Was Vicki going to retire from day placement? My experience in the past had seen people being sent off to aged care when they reached the age of 60. However, aged-care services began to show a reluctance to accept people with intellectual disabilities. I often asked what direction was going to be taken. I never received any feedback.

In March 2000 Vicki and her fellow residents were all set to enjoy their evening meal of roast pork. Details are sketchy and I don't believe we will ever know the complete facts. The evening meal was not cooked thoroughly, so large sections of the meat had been cut off and left out on the bench. The coroner's report states that both staff members sought to relieve their cigarette craving and were standing in the doorway of the patio when Vicki picked up some meat and attempted to eat it. The large portions caused Vicki to choke, and although a staff member applied CPR it was not enough to revive her and once again she suffered oxygen deprivation to her brain. While she was unconscious, she was placed on life support. After three days the doctor's prognosis for her recovery was not good and we were faced with having to make the heartbreaking decision of turning the respirator off. Our beautiful Vicki had surmounted many obstacles and difficulties in her life but this time the challenge was just too great. Our sister Vicki was gone. It just did not seem fair that she had fought and survived situations that would have defeated many others, to then lose her life in this way.

The coroner's report 12 months later did nothing to reassure me that her death had not been in vain. The coroner noted that the staff smoking policy had been broken, even though it was admitted that the policy had been reinforced two weeks earlier. I could not help coming away with the sense that justice had not been served and that Vicki's death was not of great consequence to anyone except her family. We were left to come to the painful reality that she was no longer in our lives.

Note

1 CCOR: Client Consultation on Relocation was an eight-step process implemented throughout the closure of Hilltop by which residents established their preferences for future living arrangements.

Reference

Johnson, K. (1998) *Deinstitutionalising Women: An Ethnographic Study of Institutional Closure.* Melbourne: Cambridge University Press.

16

Reflections on Living Outside

Continuity and Change in the Life of 'Outsiders'

Jan Tøssebro, Norway

What does it mean for people with intellectual disabilities to live outside institutions? There is no doubt that in some ways their lives are better. Research tells us that most people with intellectual disabilities feel good about their new lives. Families of people with intellectual disabilities sometimes do not want institutions to close but then begin to feel good about the new lives their relatives are living.

Housing people with intellectual disabilities in the community is generally better than housing them in institutions, but in important ways their lives remain similar to how they were in the institutions. For example, they do not have choices about the people with whom they live or the staff who work with them. This means that their homes are not really like those of many other adults in the community. Some people with intellectual disabilities living in the community do have the chance to work but often this does not pay a real wage; at best it adds to their pensions. So while this kind of work may be useful to them in other ways, it is not the same as the work done by many other people in the community.

Making friends can be difficult for people with intellectual disabilities living in the community. But some research tells us that they may know people who live near them, even if they are not friends.

People with intellectual disabilities living in the community do have the chance to make more day-to-day decisions about their lives than people living in institutions. But the difference is not that significant with respect to big life decisions. Sometimes this is because these kinds of decisions affect the services they use and so their views are not taken into account. Sometimes it may be because they do not know what their preferences are. It seems that some things have changed in good ways for people who have moved from institutions into the community, but in other ways their lives remain the same as they were before. Perhaps it is time to stop talking about institutions and community, and just focus on the lives of people living in the community and how they can be made better.

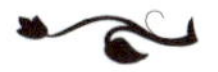

> ...the big change: I moved out of Blofield Hall. (Victor Hall, Chapter 13)

> As it turned out, my life was not much different in the community than it had been in the institution. (Thomas Allen, Chapter 12)

During the past two or three decades, many intellectually disabled people have resettled, residential institutions have been downsized or closed and a new structure of community services has emerged. One tends to say that people have 'moved out'. Even intellectually disabled people who have never been institutionalized use the phrase 'living outside' – 'outside in society' (Gustavsson 1998, pp.56–7). This chapter is about living outside. It both reflects on the four preceding chapters in Part III of this book and on experiences from 12 years of research on deinstitutionalization in Norway. My ambition is to link the two, not least since the preceding chapters illustrate typical concerns in community care. And I want to emphasize one particular concern which is reflected in the chapter title as well as the quotes above. There are definitely positive developments in community living for people with intellectual disabilities but there are also similarities to institutional life. Therefore, my theme is one of continuity and change.

A strategy commonly used to illuminate the social situation of a group of people is that of contrasts or comparisons. How are their life circumstances compared to…? The literature on people with intellectual disabilities is riddled with one such comparison: is life after relocation better or worse than in institutions? Institutions are usually seen as the 'bad old days', 'no change' is read as failure, and descriptions of 'living outside' are in reality about moving out. This is also the standpoint from which Chapters 12–15 are largely written. Another strategy, less common in studies of people with intellectual disabilities, but much more common in mainstream social research, is to compare across social groups. Women are compared to men, city folk to rural ones, single mothers to couples with children, and so on. The point is not only that such comparisons illuminate the issue at hand, but they might also serve political purposes, backing claims for action if groups are shown to be disadvantaged. Given the strong emphasis on the normalization principle in the field of disability, it is strange that this type of comparison is wanting in studies of people with intellectual disabilities 'living outside'.

The reflections in this chapter are largely based on comparisons; comparisons with life in institutions and also with non-disabled people. The issues raised are of relevance to many countries, but this chapter is nonetheless based to a large extent on Norwegian experiences. This emphasis is not only due to the fact that I am a Norwegian. Norway is among the few countries where all institutions for people with intellectual disabilities have been closed, and have been closed for nearly a decade. Thus, life 'outside' has been the dominant pattern for some time, even for people with severe intellectual (and multiple) disabilities. In Norway, too, there is a substantial body of national data on the current living conditions of people with intellectual disabilities; data which permit comparison with both institutional life and other social groups. My intention in this chapter, however, is not number-crunching but reflection. The data thus mainly serve as a background for an overall story-line, and will largely be presented indirectly as literature references (mostly Tøssebro 1996; Tøssebro and Lundeby 2002).

I do not want to suggest that all points made in this chapter are relevant across all countries and service systems. We tend to talk about institutions, deinstitutionalization and community care as if they are/were uniform phenomena, but such an assertion is imprecise, to say the least. Some institutions were huge congregations of more than 3000 people; others were local hospitals with no more than 20 residents. Some had large dormitories, others individual bedrooms. Community care is private or public; some people have their own apartments, even houses – such as Emil Johansen in Chapter 14 – others have just one private room. Tom Allen (Chapter 12) did not even have a room of his own in the community but shared it with a roommate. Given such diversity, all reflections do of course have to be tentative and approximate – they are truly reflections.

On the pages that follow I will address questions linked to the core of relocation, housing; but I will also consider neighbourhood, work and self-determination. However, let us start out with a point that is present in all the case stories: people appear to be happy about the resettlement.

Attitudes to deinstitutionalization and community care – and the problem of choice

In the early phases of deinstitutionalization, the 'movers' were typically people with a mild or moderate intellectual disability, people who spoke for themselves. All research on their point of view, with which I am familiar, suggests that people were happy about the move (for instance Birenbaum and Re 1979; Booth, Simons and Booth 1990; Edgerton and Bercovici 1976). Later, the 'movers' also included people with severe disabilities and the focus shifted to family attitudes. A fairly distinct pattern of attitudes and attitude change emerged from research with families. Briefly, families opposed resettlement prior to the fact, but were happy about it afterwards (see also Tom Allen in Chapter 12).

In a research review, Larson and Lakin (1991) found that a weighted mean of 74 per cent of the families were negative prior to relocation. In Norway, only 17 per cent thought community living would lead to improvements; a majority of 57 per cent expected a set-back (Tøssebro 1998). Fear about the results was widespread among families, and some predicted a backlash against the deinstitutionalization movement (Frohboese and Sales 1980). However, several studies, especially from the USA, did show that families changed their minds during the process. According to the review by Larson and Lakin (1991), about 60 per cent preferred the new services in the community. In Norway, about three out of four found the community services better *ex post facto*. Only 15 per cent wanted the institutions back.

This research shows that most people appear to prefer the new community services, at least after institutional closure. But since most people do not initially welcome the changes, the whole movement becomes problematic from a democratic and empowerment point of view. If users or their spokespersons had been given the power to decide, a backlash against the deinstitutionalization movement would most likely have taken place. If empowered, people would have blocked the move before they came to the point where they changed their minds.

Private territory

Deinstitutionalization (nearly) always means new accommodation. The emblem of community care is the group home. A group home is usually on a residential street and for a small group, typically three to five people, but, apart from that, variation between homes is tremendous. Some houses are purpose-built, others are not. In many cases people living in the house share the same or similar diagnoses, but there are definitely exceptions. In Norway and Sweden, residents tend to have an individual apartment with a bedroom, living room, kitchen and bathroom. The private area is usually about 50 square metres (Tideman and Tøssebro 2002). In other countries, it is more typical that people will have an individual room in an apartment shared by three to five people – some even share bedrooms. This variation between houses is partly concealed by the tendency to use one term across the field.

In spite of the variation between houses, compared to institutions, the new group homes were a significant improvement. Within the deinstitutionalization movement, housing was the 'big change'. However, the point I want to highlight here is not the improvement in housing size and standard, but the social implications of the new physical structures. One simple illustration of this can be seen in families' responses to our questionnaire (in Norway). Families were asked if they found it easier to visit their child/sibling with an intellectual disability after resettlement, and why. A large majority responded 'Yes, it is easier', and gave the reason that 'it feels more like a private visit now' (68% of the sample, Tøssebro 1996).

This illustration reflects one important, but usually taken for granted, aspect of housing: the residence as private territory. The concept of territory may sound outlandish in descriptions of people's housing. It is more often used with reference to states or animals – such as tigers and black grouse. However, in human interaction we apply a large number of rules of territoriality. We do not sit down at a café table which is already occupied, we apologize if we touch someone we pass on the street, we avoid sitting next to someone unknown on the bus unless there are no other free seats and we do not enter someone else's house unless we are invited. Moreover, these rules are not just rules but schemes for interpretation. Research on non-verbal communication has shown how we read social meaning into physical proximity (Øyslebø 1988), and there are many similarities between interaction rules and communication (Goffman 1974; Kendon, Harris and Key 1975). The communicative content when rules of territory are broken systematically is especially important in our context.

Accommodation, particularly the home, is of special significance as territory. Excluding the body, the home may pass as our core territory. It is a place where we withdraw from the public eye, where we can be our private selves. It is a place where we are supposed to be in control. Different rooms in the home are zones of privacy, with the parental bedroom being the most private. In short, our home is our castle and, as such, a territory loaded with basic instincts as well as social meaning.

Parts of the critique of institutions can be read as being about territoriality, an example being Goffman's (1961) *Asylums*. He argued that institutions invade the private area; for example, by removing personal markers and private belongings, placing people in rooms with strangers, staff entering residents' rooms without knocking on the door, and so on. Staff could even bring their own visitors into a person's room, just to show them what it was like. Thus, the living place is undermined as private territory by the operation of the institution. The 'home' thus becomes deprived of an important function, and this deprivation most likely communicates loss of dignity and status of and to participants – consciously or not.

Goffman's study was carried out at a large US psychiatric hospital in the 1950s. The typical 1980s Norwegian institution for intellectually disabled people was somewhat different but, nevertheless, people's 'homes' did appear as invaded territory (Tøssebro 1992). Some would argue that the single most important result of resettlement was about the private character of physical space. A qualitative study of the experiences of people moving into the community concluded that: 'I will never again underestimate what it means for human beings to have their own home' (S'tersdal 1994, p.77, my translation). In our own study, we included some crude indicators of the private character of accommodation, such as private domestic possessions, markers of private area (door plate, mail-box, etc.), relationships with the people in the same territory, and so on. All such indicators showed marked changes after resettlement. And all four chapters in Part III of this book (Chapters 12–15) also reflect this point.

The above argument is based on what community housing looks like if compared to institutions. But what if we change perspective and focus on deviations from the typical adult population? The typical group home is fairly different from a family home, and also from the homes of single adults. However, in Norway the National Housing Bank offered service providers favourable loans if group homes were in keeping with the principles of general housing policy. That is, the rules that the bank applied to other people were also to be applied to houses planned for people with intellectual disabilities. In the 1990s in Norway this meant, among other things, that a single-person household should have a full 'two-room' apartment (a living room and one bedroom, and also a kitchen and bathroom) of 50 square metres. Thus, in this case the principle of comparing housing for people with intellectual disabilities with that of other people came to be public policy. But of course there are also differences. In Norway, a typical family owns their house (82%) and even among single adults (20–67 years of age) the proportion is above half. Among people with intellectual disabilities it is a different story (only 11% own their own house).

However, the main point I want to discuss here is not the size or standard of housing, and so on, but the home as private territory. And, without underestimating the improvements, when compared to other people this history as it applies to people with intellectual disabilities may be written as one of continuity with institutional life. The comparison between people with intellectual disabilities and other people may seem strange and obvious, since most people do not live in group homes, but sometimes it is worthwhile reminding oneself about the obvious – because it is so easily overlooked. The most outstanding differences between people with intellectual disabilities and others are related to choice and autonomy, such as 'where shall I live?' and 'with whom?'. Even though options may be restricted for different reasons, most 'typical' people decide for themselves where to live. People with intellectual disabilities rarely do and, furthermore, neither do their advocates, legal representatives or families. In practice, housing is assigned by some authority or agency. Next to no one with an intellectual disability has any say about with whom he or she will live and for some, like Tom Allen (Chapter 12), other people's choice of a 'wrong' roommate may have severe consequences. The problem may partly reflect the very nature of group homes. People live together in a condition that is halfway between neighbours and household members, depending on the type of group home. Adult people tend to choose household members, not neighbours. In group homes, the way you live with others is largely an administrative decision by the service-providing agency. The logic of a 'free bed' prevails. The result is that your territory is not yours in the sense people usually expect.

Another important difference, which is equally obvious, is about staff support – which might very well become staff control, staff invasion or simply a lot of people coming and going. It is about professional practice, but also turnover, part-time positions, enthusiasm, and so on. In Chapter 12, Tom Allen describes his frustrations related to staff coming and going, that they appear more interested in each other than in the residents, but he also comments that one particular staff member became his 'angel'. Jen Devers, in Chapter 15, also describes staff turnover and loss of enthusiasm. I do not think there are easy ways out of this problem. To provide care and support in someone else's home requires a kind of respect and attention which may clash with the haste of a work culture and working-life boredom. During the deinstitutionalization reform in Norway, there was quite a lot of activity related to the development of staff roles to fit the new community service structure and ideology (Jensen 1992; Sandvin *et al.* 1998; Wuttudal 1994). However, it is unclear to what extent practices really changed, at least for people with extensive support needs.

These last points are not to say that changes in housing have not been a clear improvement. In Scandinavia at least they have been. The point is to remind us that there are challenges ahead, challenges we run the risk of overlooking because they are so obvious.

The new neighbourhood

Deinstitutionalization usually means relocation to a typical residential street. It is physical integration. But physical integration does not necessarily mean that people become part of their neighbourhood. Sometimes they become outcasts. During the 1980s there were many reports of opposition by local people to intellectually disabled people settling in their neighbourhood. Such reports came from very different countries, and Cnaan, Adler and Ramon (1986) are probably right when characterizing it as an international phenomenon. The big question thus became not participation, integration and inclusion, but how to avoid conflicts (see also Jen Devers, Chapter 15).

There appears to be less talk about such conflicts today. This definitely applies to Norway, but the topic is also only infrequently raised in the international research literature now. The silence seems to reflect a disappearing problem. A recent Norwegian study (Tøssebro and Lundeby 2002) found that less than 10 per cent of people with intellectual disabilities had experienced trouble with neighbours when their house was built. Given the deviant physical appearance of many group homes, the figure is actually low. My guess is that the figure would have been higher if houses with a similar appearance were for 'typical' people. People simply do not want to be associated with the image of the intolerant neighbour.

About one in eight houses for people with intellectual disabilities reports ongoing complaints or conflicts with neighbours. However, staff judged the majority of these complaints to be fair enough. They were reactions to behaviour everyone would find disturbing, and the complaints were not linked to the disability *per se*, but to specific behaviour. Therefore, it appears as if problems with neighbours are about what one would expect anywhere and for everyone. People with intellectual disabilities, as such, appear to be accepted. People are now accustomed to more diversity, both at stores and on residential streets.

Acceptance does not, however, mean integration; at least not in a social-network sense. The Norwegian case suggests variation in neighbour contacts. Some people with intellectual disabilities know neighbours well enough to ask for help or to visit them, some say 'hello, nice day' when they occasionally run into each other on the street, whereas some have no neighbour contact whatsoever. It is largely people with a mild disability who have more than superficial contact with neighbours and, according to the above-mentioned study (Tøssebro and Lundeby 2002), about 20 per cent of these people know at least one neighbour well enough to visit him/her.

It is probably not unexpected that this pattern is negative. Some people will be surprised that one in five people with intellectual disabilities really does visit neighbours occasionally. After all, modern neighbourhoods are not characterized by tight social networks. They are more like a place people pass through on their way from home to some kind of activity or business. However, people with intellectual disabilities do stand out, with fewer contacts than other people. According to the 1995 Norwegian standard of living survey,[1] a third of the population between the ages of 20 and 67 saw neighbours weekly, and the majority knew more than two neighbours well enough to visit them. One in four said they did not know any neighbours that well. In short, even if neighbourhoods are not characterized by tight social networks, most people have some contact and know some neighbour well. However, this is true for only a minority of people with intellectual disabilities.

So it appears as if acceptance and integration are different things. 'Outside', people with intellectual disabilities are accepted, but nevertheless they are still 'outside' in the social meaning of the word.

Contacts with neighbours are just a small part of most people's social network, and for people with an active network elsewhere, neighbours are of minor importance. This is not the case for most people with intellectual disabilities. Their social network seems structured according to the classical sociological concepts of ascription and achievement. At least in Norway, their social contact with family (parents and siblings) does not differ much from that of other people. These relationships are ascribed, or non-chosen, and tend to be taken for granted. But when it comes to friends, partners, neighbours and acquaintances – relationships where the aspect of choice and the achievement of a position in a network is important – then people with intellectual disabilities live in a world apart.

This account is based on a comparison between people with intellectual disabilities and 'typical' people in the community. It suggests that not much appears to have changed with their social networks during the deinstitutionalization process. Neither the 'fear of loneliness' nor the 'hope for inclusion' images appear to have come true. However, a recent Swedish study raises an aspect of social networks which is usually disregarded (Ringsby 2002). Some people with a moderate disability may not be included in social networks in the sense that they have many friends, but they do get around and live an active social life with acquaintances. The concepts of 'public places' and 'weak ties' appear to be more relevant than traditional social network concepts. Ringsby's observations also illuminate the limitations of a research strategy based on comparisons, be it with institutions or typical people. There is a risk that issues not relevant to the comparison may pass unnoticed and that innovative lifestyle patterns will remain undisclosed.

People with a more severe intellectual disability seem to be more dependent on organized activities. In that respect, community care does not seem to represent an improvement on institutions. In Norway, such activities have decreased and Tom Allen (Chapter 12) appears to have had similar experiences in the USA.

The world of work

Traditionally, people with intellectual disabilities have not taken part in the world of work. The institution was responsible for all organized activity, including the occupation of residents. There have been ups and downs in the nature and function of such work. A century ago, the agricultural, laundry and maintenance work in institutions was necessary for the running of the facility. At other times work-type activities were seen in a therapeutic perspective or simply from the view that people needed to be occupied. During the last years of institutions in Norway, a variety of work-type activities was initiated and some workshops were set up outside institution grounds. These workshops were usually intended for people with mild disabilities. The idea was that people should learn an occupation, but the workshops also separated work and home physically and underpinned an adult role for participants.

Since the famous study of unemployment in Marienthal in Austria in the 1930s (Jahoda, Lazarsfeld and Zeisel 1933), several sociological studies have discussed the social significance of work. There appears to be agreement that employment has both manifest functions, such as income, and latent functions, such as support for identity, structuring of time/everyday life, sense of purpose, social integration, social status and compliance with dominant societal values (work ethic). In short, work is an important adult role – and deprivation of that role may have serious moral costs. Given the importance for people with intellectual disabilities of holding valued social roles, the traditional valued adult role of work assumes even greater importance for this group of people (see Victor Hall's comments in Chapter 13). However, not everyone agrees with this position. Some people would argue that it is not viable to promote employment for all. Rather, we should be working to change social values in order to gain increased acceptance for alternative activities. I will not go into this discussion here, but take the importance of the work role for granted.

In most countries, adults with intellectual disabilities receive their main means of income from welfare programmes. In Norway, this comes in the form of disability pensions. However, this does not mean that people with intellectual disabilities do not work. Most of them do, but with little remuneration. The possible income from their occupation is just a supplement to their pensions. If one does not receive real wages, one's work is deprived of its core manifest function and this, in fact, changes the social meaning of work. This point is made stronger by the fact that remuneration is of minor importance even as a supplement for most people with intellectual disabilities. In Norway, only two per cent of a national sample had income from work which added 15 per cent or more to the disability benefit (Tøssebro and Lundeby 2002). Even though the implications for the meaning of work may not be absolutely clear, the flavour of unreality and pretence is discomfiting.

The lack of remuneration partly reflects the type of work in which people with intellectual disabilities are involved. Few work in competitive employment. In Norway, only four per cent of people with intellectual disabilities are involved in competitive employment. This includes people with wage subsidies, in supported employment schemes or any other programme addressing the open labour market. The majority of people with intellectual disabilities are occupied at activity centres, usually with work-type activities. A third of them are working in sheltered workshops. This is close to status quo when compared with the work of people who were in institutions.

However, the details of employment statistics are not important. The point is that deinstitutionalization has not led to the inclusion of people with intellectual disabilities in the world of work. They do work – in Scandinavia a large majority is involved in work-type activities for 20 hours or more each week. But the activities do not take place within the framework of the world of work. Even compared to other groups classified as occupationally disabled, people with intellectual disabilities stand out as not being part of inclusive labour-market programmes (Seierstad 1998).

The implications of these findings are not necessarily that the work is meaningless for people with intellectual disabilities and that they could do equally well without it. Such work structures time and everyday life. It is a safeguard against passivity. It is also a safeguard against being at home all day. For some people it may even provide some of the latent benefits of work, such as a sense of identity, a purpose and the assumption of an adult role. But it is not part of the world of work – it is a world apart. It is 'outside' – in a different way to 'outside' institutions.

Controlling my life and the zone of self-determination

All four chapters in this section of the book are in part about self-determination. Especially for Victor Hall, deinstitutionalization is about freedom and autonomy – basically speaking, about adulthood (Chapter 13). Over the last few decades, the question of self-determination or control over one's own life has gained more power in the disability field. This is true for all types of disabilities; for example, it is linked to emerging independent-living schemes and to the criticisms of professional control from people who are disabled themselves (Oliver 1996). However, this emphasis is not restricted only to disability. Core Western values, such as individual autonomy, appear to be applied to groups who traditionally have been disconnected from such values. For example, it is applied to children's rights, the 'new legalism' within psychiatry and the growing importance of the agency perspective in childhood sociology (James, Jencks and Prout 1998). This emphasis is accompanied by new professional ideals, linked to key words such as 'empowerment' and 'user participation'. With Williams, Popey and Oakley (1999), one could argue that the entire welfare sector is confronted with a new value base where the autonomy, agency and self-determination of the service user are installed.

This development also applies to intellectual disability (Wehmeyer and Meltzer 1995), particularly following deinstitutionalization. It is not straightforward to sum up experiences and research on the self-determination of people with intellectual disabilities, but the conclusions of Emerson and Hatton's 1994 UK literature review appear to provide a useful starting point (Emerson and Hatton 1994; see also Stancliffe and Abery 1997). People seem to have more self-determination after relocation from institutions, even though it is restricted compared to that of other people. However, the big problem is that the positive changes apply mainly to everyday activities, not to more important choices, such as where to live, daytime occupation, and so on. Practically speaking, service users have no choices in relation to the important decisions in their lives. These types of decisions have a potential impact on the service provider's administration and organization, acquisition of houses, staffing, and so on, and consequently the self-determination of users is overruled. (There are parallels here with the earlier discussion on territoriality.)

The Norwegian experiences are similar to those reported from the UK. People with intellectual disabilities have more say over their own everyday life in community care, but the larger and more far-reaching decisions are beyond 'the zone of self-determination'. It also seems that the main reason for more user choice in community care is linked to less 'block treatment'. Community living means that there is more freedom to take into account the needs of individuals (Tøssebro and Lundeby 2002, p.158).

The conclusion that people with intellectual disabilities have more control over their everyday life in the community than in institutions appears reliable, and it is not problematic to agree that this is an improvement. However, as a general principle it is not necessarily self-evident that more self-determination is for the better. The traditional argument for restrictions to decision-making by people with intellectual disabilities has been that many of them, in fact, need guidance and that without it they will make serious mistakes. The counter argument is basically a reference to a principle: the dignity of risk. According to this principle, mistakes are a part of individual autonomy. However, the matter is a bit more complicated than this argument suggests. The value of self-determination relates to two things:

1. the question of 'who decides'
2. the fact that only the subjects themselves have full access to their own preferences and are thus the only people in a position to really fulfil them.

The Norwegian sociologist Hernes (1975) holds that powerlessness has two distinct dimensions. You can be powerless because you are subjected to the control of other people. But you can be equally powerless if you do not know what to do to fulfil your own preferences. If you are unable to see the consequences of your own actions, is it at all clear that it is self-determination to follow your own track? If so, it is self-determination without empowerment. One runs the risk of removing the power of decision-making from those around people with intellectual disabilities only to leave them powerless to fulfil their own preferences. It is unfortunately the case that some people with intellectual disabilities would do very little if left to their own choices. Thus, self-determination can all too easily be used to withdraw services. Simpson (2001, p.113) definitely has a point when he argues that 'self-determination fits uneasily well with the reality of empty lives and little meaningful activity'.

In conclusion, I think self-determination is very important but also full of dilemmas. Not all dilemmas are solved by taking strong ideological positions or going for a one-answer-fits-all solution. I am not arguing against the need for people with intellectual disabilities to have more say in everyday activities after they leave institutions. Definitely not. I also believe strongly that the 'zone of no choice', related to where people with intellectual disabilities can work and live and with whom, needs to be challenged. Today the logic that operates in the community in relation to these decisions is very similar to the institutional one which made decisions in terms of the distribution of available 'beds'.

Institutions and community care: continuity and change

Experiences of deinstitutionalization and community care are not uniform. There is variation across countries, service providers and individuals. But cutting across all this variation, I think one very broad conclusion holds: deinstitutionalization has led to important progress. The majority of users (or their families) find services better. However, it is also clear that a lot of things have not really changed much. If we take the Norwegian case, both the changes and the continuity of deinstitutionalization can be summarized like this: with respect to major life domains, housing is much improved but, apart from that, a status quo with institutional life is a more valid description. Leisure activities have even decreased. As for individual autonomy, one can observe more self-determination in everyday activities, but not with respect to more far-reaching decisions. And the participation or inclusion of people with intellectual disabilities in social and societal life? Physical integration saw a quantum leap but, in relation to integration in working life, social networks of 'typical' people, even leisure activities, changes are modest. Socially speaking, one can observe many characteristics of people with intellectual disabilities continuing to live in a world apart. Segregation is certainly not as visible and physical as in earlier times and, even more important, it is no longer intentional. In short, there is change and continuity.

After more than 30 years of deinstitutionalization, the move out of institutions still tends to guide and also limit our thinking about services for people with intellectual disabilities. This is not just because of the community/institution, 'better/worse' comparative approach to the study of current services. The way the resettlement is established as *the* major event, the '*then*' separating before and now, is equally important. The facts may differ from country to country but, at least for Norway, the 'major event' frame is an exaggeration. By letting this 'then' overshadow the discussion, we can underestimate the significant improvements that took place inside institutions during the 1970s and 1980s, and also the continuity in many life domains after the 'move' into the community. And this emphasis underestimates the variation within types of service. Emerson and Hatton (1994, pp.25, 29), in a UK research review, have shown that group homes on average are better than hostels which again are better than hospitals. But they have also shown that the variation within types of services is as important as the variation between them.

In the longer run, the way the 'then' attracts our attention may be a limitation. Maybe it is time to discuss community care and community life on their own terms, maybe with concepts from general disability policy, such as the slogan of the UN year on disability (1981): full participation and equality.

Note

1 In some countries, including Norway, large surveys on people's standard of living (living conditions) are carried out on a regular basis (annually or more seldom). The surveys are part of the countries' social reporting/monitoring of social problems and address a wide range of life domains, such as housing, work, family life, health, social networks, income, and so on. Results from these surveys are frequently used as data sources for comparison with 'typical people'.

References

Birenbaum, A. and Re, M.A. (1979) 'Resettling mentally retarded adults in the community – almost 4 years later.' *American Journal on Mental Retardation 83*, 323–32.

Booth, T., Simons, K. and Booth, W. (1990) *Outward Bound.* Buckingham: Open University Press.

Cnaan, R., Adler, I. and Ramon, A. (1986) 'Public reactions to establishments of community residential facilities for mentally retarded persons in Israel.' *American Journal of Mental Deficiency 90*, 677–85.

Edgerton, R. and Bercovici, S. (1976) 'The cloak of competence: Years later.' *American Journal of Mental Deficiency 80*, 485–97.

Emerson, E. and Hatton, C. (1994) *Moving Out: Relocation from Hospital to Community.* London: HMSO.

Frohboese, R. and Sales, B.D. (1980) 'Parental opposition to deinstitutionalisation.' *Law and Human Behavior 12*, 1–87.

Goffman, E. (1961) *Asylums.* New York: Doubleday.

Goffman, E. (1974) *Frame Analysis.* New York: Harper & Row.

Gustavsson, A. (1998) *Inifrån utanförskapet* ('Inside the outsider's perspective'). Stockholm: Johansson & Skyttmo.

Hernes, G. (1975) *Makt og avmakt* ('Power and powerlessness'). Oslo: Universitetsforlaget.

Jahoda, M., Lazarsfeld, P. and Zeisel, H. (1933) *Die Arbeitslosen von Marienthal.* ('Marienthal: The sociography of an unemployed community'). London: Tavistock.

James, A., Jencks, C. and Prout, A. (1998) *Theorizing Childhood.* Cambridge: Polity Press.

Jensen, K. (1992) *Hjemlig omsorg i offentlig regi* ('Home-based services and public management'). Oslo: Universitetsforlaget.

Kendon, A., Harris, R. and Key, M. (eds) (1975) *Organization of Behavior in Face-to-face Interaction.* The Hague: Mouton Publishers.

Larson, S.A. and Lakin, K.C. (1991) 'Parent attitudes about residential placement before and after deinstitutionalization: A research synthesis.' *Journal of the Association for Persons with Severe Handicaps 16*, 25–38.

Oliver, M. (1996) *Understanding Disability.* London: Macmillan.

Øyslebø, O. (1988) *Ikke-verbal kommunikasjon* ('Non-verbal communication'). Oslo: Universitetsforlaget.

Ringsby-Jansson, B. (2002) *Vardagslivets Arenor* ('Arenas of everyday life'). Gothenburg: Gothenburg University.

Sætersdal, B. (1994) *Menneskeskjebner i HVPU-reformens tid* ('Human fortunes in the era of deinstitutionalization'). Oslo: Universitetsforlaget.

Sandvin, J., Söder, M., Lichtwarck, W. and Magnussen, T. (1998) *Normalisering og Ambivalens* ('Normalisation and ambivalence'). Oslo: Universitetsforlaget.

Seierstad, S. (1998) 'Utsyn over statlige og kommunale attføringstiltak' ('Review of labour market programmes for people with occupational disabilities'). In S. Seierstad, A.K. Eide, K.M. Helle and A. Schaft (eds) *Evaluering av de statlige arbeidssamvirketiltakene og de kommunale aktivitetstilbudene for yrkeshemmede* ('Evaluating State and municipal labour market programmes'). Oslo: AFIs rapportserie 5/98.

Simpson, M. (2001) 'Programming adulthood: Intellectual disability and adult services.' In D. May (ed.) *Transition and Change in the Lives of People with Intellectual Disabilities.* London: Jessica Kingsley Publishers.

Stancliffe, R. and Abery, B. (1997) 'Longitudinal study of deinstitutionalisation and the exercise of choice.' *Mental Retardation 35*, 159–69.

Tideman, M. and Tøssebro, J. (2002) 'A comparison of living conditions for intellectually disabled people in Norway and Sweden: Following the national reforms in the 1990s.' *Scandinavian Journal of Disability Research 4*, 23–42.

Tøssebro, J. (1992) *Institusjonsliv i velferdsstaten* ('Institutions in the welfare state'). Oslo: ad Notam Gyldendal.

Tøssebro, J. (1996) *En bedre hverdag? Utviklingshemmetes levekår etter HVPU-reformen* ('A better life? Intellectually disabled people's living conditions after relocation from institutions'). Oslo: Kommuneforlaget.

Tøssebro, J. (1998) 'Family attitudes to deinstitutionalisation before and after resettlement: The case of a Scandinavian welfare state.' *Journal of Developmental and Physical Disabilities 10*, 55–72.

Tøssebro, J. and Lundeby, H. (2002) *Statlig reform og kommunal hverdag: Utviklingshemmetes levekår ti år etter reformen* ('State reform and local practice: Living conditions of intellectually disabled people ten years after resettlement'). Trondheim: Norwegian University of Science and Technology.

Wehmeyer, M. and Metzler, C. (1995) 'How self-determined are people with mental retardation? The national consumer survey.' *Mental Retardation 33*, 111–119.

Williams, F., Popey, J. and Oakley, A. (1999) *Welfare Research: A Critical Review.* London: UCL Press.

Wuttudal, K. (1994) *Tjenesteyting i boliger til psykisk utviklingshemmete* ('Services in group homes for people with intellectual disabilities'). Trondheim: Allforsk.

PART IV

Moving On

17

A New Life

Thomas F. Allen
with Rannveig Traustadóttir and Lisa Spina, USA

My life in the apartment is much better since Lisa started working with me. She helps me with everything I want to do. We read the paper in the morning and when the weather is good we go out. We go downtown, go shopping, visit different places and have lunch at a restaurant. In the summer we go to the beach, for a picnic or on boat rides on the Finger Lakes. Lisa also helps me go fishing, which I like very much.

I have been fighting against institutions and took part in a public forum to close Syracuse Developmental Center. I wrote a statement based on my experiences of institutions. I described how bad the institutions had been and said I had felt like I was in a prison being punished like a criminal and all I had was a disability.

It was in many ways good living in the apartment, but it was not a real home. I was getting old and wanted to have a real home before I died. I wanted to live with a family in a real home. I asked many people to help me but we could not find a home for me. I became very sick and was in the hospital. They wanted to put me into a nursing home. I had spent enough time in institutions and did not want to go back. I decided I wanted to go back home to the apartment. I did not want to die in an institution.

I lived in institutions for 60 years and I often felt I lived for nothing. This is the reason I want to tell my story. I want to leave something behind. No one should have to go through what I have been through. I want my story to be a lesson in how *not* to treat anyone, disabled or non-disabled. This is why I want to tell my story.

Tom Allen's story is continued from Chapter 12. Please see pp.34–35 and the Epilogue to Thomas F. Allen's Life Story on p.274 for a description of how the story was told and written.

Tom's story *continued*

Every day Lisa and I begin by reading the morning paper. If it is nice out we go wherever we want to but on days when it rains we do my laundry and read a book. At 1.30 every day I check the mail and sometimes there is a letter for me. Lisa reads my mail to me and helps me write back to my friends and relatives. Every Friday I sit down and look at next week's menu and decide what I want to eat. Then Lisa and I make up our own special grocery list and we go and buy things I can eat. Sometimes we also buy things I should not eat. Because of my stomach problems I should stay away from certain things but sometimes we ignore that and buy things I like, even if they are not good for me. It might not seem very important to some people to be able to decide what you eat. For years I had no choice about my food. Now I can finally make decisions. It is very important to me.

Every day Lisa and I pick a place to go. Sometimes we need the van and sometimes we walk. We walk around downtown Syracuse, for example to the Galleries, a great new shopping mall, where I go to the library for books and VCR movies. I often stop in the music store to look at tapes. I often have lunch at the Galleries and sometimes my friends meet me for lunch at one of the fast-food restaurants. And we sometimes go to the bakery in the Galleries for goodies, especially chocolate éclairs, my favourite.

We are also within walking distance of the post office, book stores, the Salvation Army, the Wagon Wheel – which is a pretty little place where Lisa reads aloud to me – and a few ice-cream stores. Lisa also helps me take care of my finances and she takes me to the drugstore for things I need. A few times a year we also go shopping for shoes and clothing. Sometimes we go downtown and sometimes we take the van and go to shopping malls. Lisa takes me to doctors' appointments and helps me keep track of my medication. I take medication for my asthma and my stomach.

We go to the beach in the summer and Lisa helps me go fishing which I enjoy very much. We take boat rides on the Finger Lakes, go camping, go on picnics and to the Farmers' Market. If I want to talk to some of the agency people, Lisa drives me over there in the van and helps me talk to them.

Lisa helps me call my friends and family on the phone, and a couple of times a year she takes me to see my brother Neal and my sister Marion. Both live a few hours' drive from Syracuse but in opposite directions so I cannot visit both of them in the same trip. And Lisa helps me go to the family reunion every year. I have a large family and I love to see all my nephews and nieces.

At night or on weekends I sometimes go to the movies or to a show or a play at the Landmark Theater. I enjoy very much going to the State Fair and sometimes I go a couple of times each year. I also go to parties. We have birthday celebrations for all the residents in my apartment, the other apartments and group homes the agency runs. They are fun. My favourite party of all was my retirement party.

Fighting against institutions

Some of my friends started a coalition to close Syracuse Developmental Center (SDC) and there was an 'Open Forum to Close Syracuse Developmental Center' which was held downtown Syracuse in the Legislative Chambers in the Onondaga County's Court House. A friend asked me to make a statement to the open forum and I put together a statement based on my experiences in institutions. One of the staff members took me over there. The Legislative Chambers were packed with people. People had to stand in the hallways because they could not get in. Some of the people who were there had disabilities and had lived in institutions. Most of them had moved out like me but some still lived in institutions. The open forum was very powerful. A number of people with disabilities gave statements and testimonies about how it was to live in institutions and why they should be closed. Many people without disabilities also gave speeches and said SDC should be closed. When it was my turn to give my statement the staff woman who was with me read it for me. I cannot speak clearly enough myself. The statement is as follows:

> I have been in three different institutions in 60 years. If I had my way I would close every damn institution in the United States.
>
> Living in an institution is Hell. You never know what is going to happen to you. I have seen people die for no reason. I have seen people get punished for no reason. I am one of them. I have been put in a corner, facing the wall, for hours on end simply for talking out of line.
>
> To me all institutions are alike. One might be a little better than the other but not by much.
>
> - You cannot do what you want to do.
> - You have no freedom.
> - You have no respect.
> - You have no dignity.
> - You have very few friends.
>
> What few friends I did have I needed to be very careful what I said not to get myself or them in trouble.
>
> In some places I have lived there have been bed bugs, cockroaches – anything unsanitary.
>
> Moving out was the greatest day of my life. I have been going places and doing things I have always wanted to. In order for me to get out of the institution I had to get a lawyer and fight in court for my freedom and for the freedom of others.
>
> I felt like I was in a prison being punished like a criminal and all I had was a disability.
>
> I want everybody with a disability to be free as much as possible in this country.

When she had read my statement, I said a few words. People applauded for a long time after my statement. It made me feel good. I really want to do my share to close SDC and all other institutions.

A home before I die?

My life changed when Lisa started working with me. For the first time in my life I could do the things I had always wanted to do. She and I became very close friends. I consider her to be my best friend and she knows me better than anybody else. With her help I regained my hope and desire to live.

On 9 March 1990 I quietly celebrated my fifth anniversary living in the community. I have learned something new about myself during the past five years. Living in the apartment has helped me see that I have the right to speak up for what I want and that my feelings are important and they count.

Still, the apartment is not a real home and I would like to have a home before I die. In October 1989 I decided I wanted to leave the apartment and move in with a family and have a real home. I did not tell anyone but Lisa at first but we soon began working on making this happen.

We went over to the agency's office and talked to the person who is in charge of Family Care. We explained my situation and she said she would help me find a family I could live with. I did a newspaper article and ran a couple of ads in Pennysavers. The people who responded did not seem to be the right people for me to live with. I also got nice letters from people who read the article and wished me luck in finding a home. This was not working out as well as I had hoped so I went to another agency which does Family Care and asked them to also help me find a home. I figured that the more places that knew what I wanted the better my chances for getting a home.

Because things were not working out we decided to have a meeting with some of my friends to try to see if they could come up with better ways of finding a family for me to live with. After that meeting we distributed flyers with my picture in churches and other places we thought would be frequented by people I would like to live with.

The months passed and nothing happened but I was still hopeful I would find a home before I died. Then, in January of 1991, I got very sick and was in the hospital for ten days. I had renal failure. The doctors gave me two options: to get dialysis and go into a nursing home or go home and spend what time I had left there, without dialysis.

I needed dialysis to live. My kidneys were not functioning properly but the only way I could get dialysis was if I went into a nursing home. If I did not have dialysis I would not be able to live very long. I decided not to go to a nursing home. I had spent enough of my life in institutions and I will never enter one again to live there. I decided to go home.

Suddenly, when I was faced with the threat of being put in an institution, the apartment did not seem all that bad. It was the closest to home I had experienced since I was a child. It was certainly a better place to die than an institution. I wanted to die at home.

I was becoming quite weak and fragile and had to go back into the hospital four weeks later. This time I had pneumonia and stayed in the hospital for a week.

The doctors did not think I would make it this time but I did. I still don't know what keeps me going. I felt very helpless and insecure in the hospital because I could not call the nurses if I needed anything or if something happened. During both of these hospital stays my friends and some of the staff from the apartments stayed with me so I was never alone. They even took turns staying overnight. It was very comforting having them there.

During my long stay in the institution I missed my family very much. I felt lonely and isolated. I did not want to be locked up away from everything and everybody. I wanted to be a part of the world and wanted to leave the institution. I dreamed about the things I would do when I left. I dreamed of having a wife and children. I longed for a family: my own family like my brothers and sisters had. A happy family like we had been before my mother died. What I wanted most of all was to have a wife; a woman that I loved and who loved me back. This dream was what kept me going. It kept me alive. During times of despair I turned to it and it comforted me and gave me strength. I have held on to this dream all my life and never stopped hoping it would come true.

I have always thought of myself as an ordinary person. I wanted to lead a normal life and have a family. My life, however, was not meant to be that way and turned out to be quite different. Because of my disability, I have spent 60 years in institutions, isolated from the people I loved and unable to live the kind of life I longed for. Many times I have asked myself: 'Why did this have to happen to me?'

Much of my life has been wasted and I am sometimes overwhelmed by the feeling that I have lived for nothing. This is the reason I want to tell my story. I want to leave something behind. I am neither angry nor bitter and I don't want to blame anyone for how my life turned out. But no one should have to go through what I have been through. If my life can be a lesson in how *not* to treat anyone – disabled or non-disabled – I have accomplished something important. Then I have left something behind and my life has not been completely wasted. This is the reason I want to tell my story.

It has taken me a long time to write this story. I started writing it while I was in the institution. I had nothing to do with my time and started it to have something to do. The long days, weeks, months and years of nothingness in the institution are very difficult and having the story to work on helped me survive. Now, at the age of 78, my life is coming to its end and I want to finish the story before I die.

Tom Allen's story concludes in the Epilogue on p.274.

18

Conquering Life

The Experiences of the First Integrated Generation

Magnus Tideman, Sweden

In Sweden, all institutions for people with intellectual disabilities have been closed. Children and young people with intellectual disabilities live at home with their parents and go to the same schools as other children. Adults with intellectual disabilities live in the same kind of houses as other adults. These people, who have always lived at home and been part of their local communities, are sometimes called 'the first integrated generation'. They are the first generation who has never had to live in institutions. When they were growing up there were no institutions in their country, Sweden.

Integration into the community is good in many ways but it can also cause some problems. This chapter deals, for example, with the difficulties adults with mild intellectual disabilities have in making friends with adults who are not intellectually disabled.

Meeting other people who are in similar situations helps one find the strength to make a better life for oneself. One can do this at a meeting place for people with intellectual disabilities. There people can meet and discuss what is going well and what is difficult in their lives. They can also do things together. 'Integrated life' is good in many ways but sometimes one needs the support of others in order to make life good enough.

Case study: Anna

Anna is a young woman with Down's syndrome. She grew up with her parents, brother and sister. During her childhood she went to the same preschool and compulsory school as children without disabilities. Today Anna lives in her own apartment in an ordinary residential quarter. She thinks that, as an adult, she lives a good life in many ways. She is independent and makes her own decisions about her everyday life and how she spends her time. Anna works in a cafeteria. During working hours she meets other people who, like herself, have an intellectual disability. But she also meets people without disabilities in the cafeteria. She feels that people take her and her opinions seriously, and that she is mostly treated with respect, even if it often takes Anna a little longer, for example, to add up the price of three coffees and two cookies.

Anna thinks it is obvious that she needs support from time to time in different ways. She enjoys using different technical aids and finds them a great help when it comes to things such as telling the time. But she also needs human services and support. Personal support is necessary to ensure that Anna's everyday life proceeds without too many problems and to enable her to take part in all the exciting and enjoyable events life has to offer. During weekends and evenings Anna participates in an organization which has music and singing as its main activities. She meets a lot of people during these activities, both with and without disabilities. In many ways Anna is living an active and meaningful life, a life in which she experiences the same challenges and possibilities as other people in society.

Anna is part of what is often called 'the first generation of integration' (Gustavsson 1999). This includes the first generation of children and young people with intellectual disabilities, who have, just like non-disabled children, spent their childhood with their parents, in mainstream schools, in ordinary society. Members of this generation are the first for 150 years who have not had to live in institutions as the first alternative. The development since the 1960s of a disability policy characterized by deinstitutionalization and the ambition to offer normal living conditions to people with disabilities has had many positive results. Due to the closure of institutions and increase in open services and supports, people with intellectual disabilities can enjoy and experience many advantages in their ordinary life today. But there are exceptions and one of these is Claes.

Case study: Claes

Many years ago, when I was a teenager, I met Claes at a youth centre in Helsingborg. We were almost the same age and had a lot in common: we both lived with our parents but wanted to leave home, and we were both in our last year at school and longed to work and make money. Most of our waking time was spent contemplating life, not least love. We both wanted to meet beautiful girls, have sexual experiences and 'conquer life'.

Claes was big, strong and outgoing, while I was tall, thin and a bit shy. Of the two of us, Claes should have been the one with the best chance of success with the girls, but that was not how it turned out. Claes had a mild intellectual disability. His disability was not visible or noticeable at first meeting. But when conversations moved to uncharted territories, when a capacity for abstract thinking was required, Claes's ability fell short. And when his ability faltered he tried to compensate by becoming loud and boastful. When the girls realized that all was not right they backed off. Claes was abandoned time and again, and almost every time he came to me and asked why.

Claes sensed he was different and that after a while girls would become a little afraid of him or assume a superior attitude. What was going on? What could he do about it? Soon Claes found a way of dealing with the situation. Next time there was a disco at the youth centre, he brought a bottle of wine and some beer. When he drank alcohol the feeling of being different disappeared and he made many friends. Both girls and boys wanted to spend time with him and Claes happily treated everyone to drinks.

A few years later I ran into Claes in the city centre. He was unkempt, worn out and discontented. He told me he had gradually begun to drink more and more often. An increasing number of situations required a 'little something' beforehand. Many people desired his company but after a while he discovered they were only interested in the alcohol, not in him as a person.

The friends Claes made had problems themselves, both with alcohol and other issues, but he was welcome among them, at least if he had money or alcohol, or helped them with petty break-ins. Claes's dream of having a normal life with a job, family and independent housing had been shattered. The last time I met Claes he was waiting to serve his first prison term.

The first integrated generation

The progress made in Sweden over the past 30–40 years for people with intellectual or other disabilities is closely linked with the growth and development of the welfare state. The Swedish, or Scandinavian, welfare developments during the 1960s and 1970s involved reforms that aimed to create a better life for all citizens, gradually also including people with disabilities. Towards the end of the 1960s the concepts 'normalization' and 'integration' became the guiding stars of disability policies. Institutional life was increasingly criticized and so-called 'care in the community' was supported as an alternative.

Gradually, a growing number of people began to agree that children with disabilities were better off living with their biological parents, attending the same preschools as other children, receiving their education in the same schools and living in the same residential areas as other people. People with disabilities were no longer to be segregated but integrated into the community. Claes, in the example above, is a representative, albeit not an average one, of the first generation of people with intellectual disabilities who grew up with their parents and lived in normal residential areas, a generation in which almost no one was physically segregated or placed in an institution.

Today all institutions for people with disabilities in Sweden have been closed down and all people with intellectual disabilities below the age of 40, like Claes, have lifelong experience of living within the local community. On the one hand, this development has led today to people with intellectual disabilities living and going to school with non-disabled people, being visible in most parts of society without causing any noticeable reaction from those around them and approaching the same standard of living as the rest of society enjoys (Tideman 2000). On the other hand, the expectation that physical integration would automatically lead to social integration has not been met. Research and evaluations of integration show that people with intellectual disabilities seldom develop any deep or prolonged social relations with people without intellectual disabilities. They live in the local community, physically close to others, but without any close contact. Therefore, our experience reveals many positive effects of the development of normalization and integration, which are discussed in other chapters of this book, but also the difficulties of following through the integration completely.

In this chapter I highlight and focus on a particular group of people with intellectual disabilities: young adults with mild intellectual disabilities. This group has grown up fully physically integrated in every way. In their daily lives they have, perhaps more clearly than any other group, experienced the pros and cons of integration.

The right to participate despite difficulties

Physical proximity to 'normal people' does not necessarily imply that people with intellectual disabilities automatically have social contact with them. There is a risk that while people are physically integrated, they remain largely socially segregated (Rönsen-Ekeberg 1995). Integrated people's opportunities for social contact with 'normal people' have not noticeably been affected by their physical integration (Gustavsson 1999). People can live as neighbours for years without breaking the barrier of alienation (Daun 1980). Most people seek out the people they like best or with whom they have most in common. Similarity creates a feeling of security. People do not perceive this as excluding anyone, but take choosing one's own company for granted. This means that there are few people without intellectual disabilities in the personal networks around people with intellectual disabilities. Consequently, some people claim that for the first integrated generation social integration has failed and point out that for most people, such as Claes, integration leads to loneliness and misery.

Modern social life has become increasingly focused on the individual, and most social situations (except the family) are based on choice. This further increases the risk that those who are perceived as different will be excluded and treated differently. In spite of this, studies such as Gustavsson's (1999) of the first integrated generation in Sweden show that people with intellectual disabilities in the first integrated generation have developed faith in their right to participate in all social events and to be respected like other people, even when they have experienced disparagement and exclusion. One might have assumed that people with intellectual disabilities would give up in their attempts at participating in society on the same terms as everyone else as a result of their disability and negative experiences of social exclusion. Instead, many people with intellectual disabilities have developed an image of themselves as normal human beings with certain weaknesses or problems. In their perception such difficulties mean only that it is sometimes hard for them to meet high performance demands and because of this they have the right to support from those around them. They often avoid the disparaging label 'intellectually disabled' but at the same time want to secure the support their difficulties require. They claim the right to be accepted as they are and to be given support when they need it, even though they live in a society which in many ways upholds ideals that exclude people with reduced intellectual capacity.

Meeting Place No. 10

The old institutions robbed people with intellectual disabilities of experiences. Sadly, this is to some extent still the case in society at large. The concern of parents or health-care professionals, who wish to plan the lives of the first integrated generation of young adults with mild intellectual disabilities, can act as a barrier that hinders these people from having their own experiences. The challenge facing us is to avoid institutional care, while also avoiding the social isolation which may take its place. The well-meaning care and concern of service providers or families can devalue the very opportunities for experience and development that living in the community offers.

> Before a trip to Denmark, Kalle, in his 40s, was given many admonitions. His family and carers had told him he was not allowed to do this and that. For example, according to them he was unable to handle money and could not cope with drinking beer. During the trip his behaviour was faultless. On the last day he bought some beer, like the rest of the holiday group. Kalle was walking along the shopping street with the bottle in his hand enjoying life when suddenly he met a woman who fixed her eyes on him. It was one of the carers from Kalle's day centre. Her first comment was: 'What do you have in your hand?' Kalle's smile faded. He was ashamed, became anxious and felt as if he had been caught red-handed. It was frightening to see how quickly he was transformed from a happy 40-year-old man to a browbeaten, scared little boy. (Svensson and Lundgren 2002, p.24)

Like Kalle and Claes, many people with mild intellectual disabilities can easily become outsiders in their communities. On the one hand, they are expected to cope on their own, despite their sometimes limited capacity for taking the initiative. On the other, they are not considered to have sufficient knowledge to cope with all the situations they encounter. They do not require long-term or extensive support, but their support needs vary according to the situation or occasion. However, the support provided by the community is seldom flexible but often confined by the resources allocated and influenced by traditional views. In order to be able to shape new and different identities and to be allowed to experience their own opportunities and difficulties, these people often need to be able to meet others in the same or similar situations. Meeting Place No. 10 is an example of a place where people who share the fact of being regarded as different can attempt to make normal lives for themselves (Svensson and Lundgren 2002). Arranging this meeting place for young adults with intellectual disabilities was an attempt to help and support them in their efforts to conquer their lives.

Meeting Place No. 10 was a building in the centre of town that was open a couple of evenings a week. Most people who went to No. 10 were deeply unhappy about their situation; they felt devalued and excluded. Many of them dreamt of transforming their lives but sensed no real support for this from the people around them. The most common theme during the popular discussion evenings concerned the assumption of responsibility and respect. They listened to each other and shared their experiences. It was an unusual and very satisfying experience to have others listening to what they had to say and this became an important informal support in everyday life. Participating in group activities expanded their horizons. One way of gaining knowledge about life and a new identity is to try things out: 'learning by doing'. The individual goal for participants at Meeting Place No. 10 was to shape, with the help of others, a coherent life story and to assume the lead role in this process, with the chance of influencing its development. The group also aimed to gain a collective awareness through their shared experiences. This collective disability awareness was not based on individual recognition of deficiency but on learning to demand respect for oneself from the community.

The importance of weak ties

> Svante is visiting a town in south Sweden. After eating a hot dog and looking around the shops it is time to go home again. Svante walks towards the bus stop. The bus has not arrived yet. Svante, who cannot read the names of the destinations on the buses, nor orientate himself with the aid of bus numbers, approaches the wrong bus. Before his companion has time to intervene, a bus driver notices him and calls:
>
> 'Hey Svante, it's the wrong bus, because you're going home, aren't you?'
>
> 'Yes, I'm going home,' replies Svante, a little confused.
>
> 'Then just wait here a minute and the bus you should take will arrive; wait there and I'll tell you when the bus comes,' says the driver. Svante waves a thank you and waits, secure in the knowledge that the driver will make sure he gets on the right bus. (Ringsby-Jansson 2002, p.221)

Those who criticize integration and highlight the social isolation of some people with disabilities often do not appreciate the so-called 'weak ties' that many people with intellectual disabilities develop. The immediate neighbourhood is an area where many people with intellectual disabilities have important, albeit not very intense, relationships with, for example, the hairdresser, caretaker, restaurant owner, shopkeeper or bus driver, as in the case of Svante (Ringsby-Jansson 2002). These relationships are of great importance for everyday social life and represent important aspects of social integration. It is also common for critics to ignore the contact people with intellectual disabilities have with each other. These contacts are 'not counted'; they are not regarded as good enough or of significant value.

Treatment on different levels

Self-respect and the right to be an equal citizen are closely associated with the questions of treatment and attitudes. The right to be a citizen on equal terms implies that people who have some form of disability have the right to full participation in society. This presumes that each individual is respected and treated with dignity, and given the means of taking control of his or her own life. In order for people with intellectual disabilities to realize this right, the treatment of them needs to be improved. Treatment is defined by more than the individual meeting between the person with a disability and a public official. The treatment of someone is usually described as a system on three levels – collective, organizational and individual (SOU 1999). These levels are of course interdependent. The collective level highlights society's view of people with disabilities, expressed chiefly through national policies and legislation. The organizational level consists of how disability policies and legislation are interpreted on a local level; for example, how support is organized and how much money is allocated to various support programmes. The individual level concerns the contact between the person with a disability and the representative of society; for example, in the shape of a school or social worker. In this meeting, the values, intentions and insight of the individual official are of great importance as to how the treatment is perceived and to how disability policies are made concrete.

A research conference held in Sweden in 1999 (FUB 1999) was probably the first of its kind in the world. It is an isolated example of how the treatment of people with disabilities can be developed and improved for the first integrated generation in particular. The conference brought together academics from various disciplines and people with intellectual disabilities. The conference took place on the terms of the people with intellectual disabilities and the academics were 'forced' to present and discuss their findings in a way that was accessible to those really concerned.

Threats to integration

In Sweden today we can see a development where, although integration and participation are political goals and visions, the segregation of support efforts for some people with disabilities is becoming increasingly common. The fact that a growing number of children is categorized as having an intellectual disability or given neuro-psychiatric diagnoses is an example of this trend. The reason for this is debatable. In simplified terms, some suggest that this development is due to real individual difficulties that have only recently been discovered and named, while others argue that the problems caused by severe funding cuts in Swedish schools during the 1990s have led to significantly reduced levels of support for under-performing students (Tideman 2000).

Regardless of the reasons, the increasing categorization of children leads to further efforts at segregation, particularly within schools. For example, it is becoming increasingly common to separate children from the rest of their class, and health-care and psychology experts are suggesting the need for special classes and schools. The boundaries defining who is normal are slowly being moved in conjunction with this increasing categorization and as a result the number of people with disabilities is growing. This development partly threatens the ideas of integration and inclusion, and it could be said that today the matter hangs in the balance. Should the vision of integration continue, undergo modification or even be replaced by the school of thought which suggests that segregation is in the interests of people with disabilities? As I see it, what happens in the future is largely dependent on the financial conditions for schools and care for people with disabilities. The less money, the more segregation; the more money, the more inclusion.

Conquering the world

The Scandinavian welfare state, which has dominated progress during the lives of the integrated generation, was founded upon the fundamental idea that it is possible and desirable to create a good life for everyone. Everybody, regardless of disabilities or other difficulties, should through various social reforms enjoy a decent and meaningful life. The right to normal living conditions and normalization was seen as necessary in order for people with disabilities to be integrated into the community. In the Scandinavian countries, plans for normalization and integration have been implemented through the closure of institutions for people with disabilities and the expansion of the education, support and services available to them in the local community. This development has brought about a great deal of good but also some problems. People with intellectual disabilities have been given access to ordinary environments such as schools and residential neighbourhoods. Both integrating and segregating influences are present in these environments. 'Normal life' brings numerous advantages but also disadvantages. The first integrated generation has experienced many benefits, but some, such as Claes, have also experienced 'the flip side of the coin'.

One problem that people with disabilities face is the demand to change and adapt to society: to become normalized. Being oneself is not good enough. Out of that feeling the need has grown for people with disabilities to spend time with others like themselves, people who have the same kind of problems without this being regarded as a failure. In recent years, organizations exclusively for people with intellectual disabilities have appeared and programmes such as Meeting Place No. 10 now fulfil an important role for the first integrated generation. Programmes of this kind can be seen as parallel with, for example, women's self-help groups or lesbian and gay groups. The new organizations and meeting places are the foundations of a movement that demands participation and equality, criticizes the dominant role of health-care professionals in the care of people with disabilities, and objects to inaccessibility and discrimination in society. It can be regarded as a movement that is founded on the right to be oneself, and the equal right of everyone to participate in society. This right also includes being allowed to spend time with others like oneself if one so chooses, in order to gain strength, find security and discuss life's difficulties. Fundamentally, this resembles the so-called 'relative concept of disability', which dictates that the environment and surroundings should be adapted to people with disabilities rather than the other way round. The right of everyone to participate in the different levels of society demands that society considers and adapts to people's abilities.

Living in the community, being integrated and participating in it, has many advantages not highlighted in this chapter. However, in order for these advantages to be realized, it is also necessary for people with intellectual disabilities to receive support from, and exchange experiences with, others in similar situations, as well as receiving flexible and individually adapted support from society. It is a question of giving people with intellectual disabilities help and support, so that they can conquer their own lives, as well as the world: 'Drinking water from a mountain creek in Norway or beer at a festival in Denmark is not only about quenching thirst but also about conquering the world...' (Svensson and Lundgren 2002, p.3).

References

Daun, Å. (1980) *Livsform och boende* ('Housing and ways of life'). Stockholm: Tiden.

FUB (1999) *FUB's research conference 10–11 June 1999: A meeting between researchers and people with learning disabilities.* Stockholm: FUB.

Gustavsson, A. (1999) *Inifrån utanförskapet* ('From within the outsidership'). Lund: Studentlitteratur.

Ringsby-Jansson, B. (2002) *Vardagslivets arenor. Om människor med utvecklingsstörning, deras vardag och sociala liv* ('Arenas of everyday life: About people with intellectual disabilities and their everyday and social life'). Göteborg: Institutionen för socialt arbete, Göteborgs universitet.

Rönsen-Ekeberg, T. (1995) *Tanker og forskning om integrering av psykiskt utviklingshemmede* ('Thoughts and research on the integration of the intellectually disabled'). Monografi 23. Jaren: Skolepsykologi.

SOU (1999) *Lindqvists nia: Nio vägar att utveckla bemötandet av funktionshindrade* ('Lindqvist's Nine: Nine ways of developing the treatment of disabled people'). Stockholm: SOU.

Svensson, O. and Lundgren, K. (2002) *Mötesplats 10:an – rapport om en social försöksverksamhet, en mötesplats för unga vuxna med lindrig utvecklingsstörning* ('Meeting Place No. 10: A report on a social experiment, a meeting place for young adults with mild intellectual disabilities'). Halmstad: Wigforssgruppen & FUB utveckling.

Tideman, M. (2000) *Normalisering och kategorisering: Om handikappideologi och välfärdspolitik i teori och praktik för personer med utvecklingsstörning* ('Normalization and categorization: About disability ideology and welfare policies in theory and practice for people with intellectual disabilities'). Lund: Studentlitteratur.

19

New Forms of Institutionalization in the Community

Julian Gardner and Louise Glanville, Australia

Deinstitutionalization has had very positive effects for many people with intellectual disabilities in Victoria, Australia. As part of the movement of people into community living, people's rights have been protected and supported by laws. The hope was that people with intellectual disabilities would be able to live free and ordinary lives in the community and receive support when they needed it.

However, moving into the community has sometimes meant that people lead lives which are not free. Jason has an intellectual disability and lived in the community. He has abused small children and was imprisoned for this. Because people were anxious that he might abuse other children, a guardian was appointed for him to make decisions about his accommodation and health. As a result, Jason has been living in a secure facility for two years where he is receiving treatment. In the past, Jason would have lived in an institution. Now he lives in an institution-like place in the community.

Maria lives in a group home in the community. However, because some of the people she lives with wander away, the doors are locked. Maria therefore has less freedom than she would like or should have.

Also, staff time that could be used to support her is being used to support people with higher needs. She is living in a locked place from which the community is excluded. So, while for many people deinstitutionalization has led to more freedom, for some it has led to new kinds of institutions in the community.

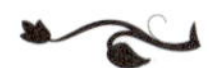

The process of deinstitutionalization in Victoria, Australia is one that is very similar in its description and timing to the process in many other parts of the world. The closure of large and not-so-large residential institutions began in 1984. Now only three large institutions remain open out of those which had for many years been home for thousands of people with an intellectual disability or a mental illness (or others with misdiagnosed conditions). The largest of these remaining facilities is undergoing a gradual process of closure which was announced in May 2001.

Many of the people moving out of institutions in Victoria (or younger people who have never moved into them) now live in suburban houses which accommodate four to five people and which are staffed on a 24-hour basis. In Victoria these are known as community residential units. Those living in the units range from people with quite profound disabilities to others who enjoy varying levels of interaction with the community. The units are run either by the government or by non-government agencies which are contracted by the government. Other people who were once in institutions now live independently in their own flats or houses with varying levels of support that is not provided on a 24-hour basis. Others again live with their families with some support services made available to facilitate this.

For most people who moved out of the large congregate-care institutions into residential settings in the community, the move has been a positive one. However, there are those for whom deinstitutionalization has meant a move to a different form of accommodation that has some or all of the features of an institution. At worst there are those who continue to experience restrictions upon their freedom of movement and other freedoms of decision-making. At best there are those whose individual needs have not been addressed.

Critical to the successful transition is the availability of a variety of forms of accommodation with appropriate levels of support; staff with sufficient knowledge, skills and motivation and the possibility of individuals making choices. Deficiencies in the law have in some cases also created restrictions on liberty.

Before looking at two case studies, it is useful to note that accompanying the new policies on institutional closure were a number of new laws passed by parliament that were designed to protect the rights of people with disabilities. These included the Intellectually Disabled Persons' Services Act 1986, the Mental Health Act 1986 and the Guardianship and Administration Act 1986. These laws set out principles to govern the provision of services to people with an intellectual disability. These included promoting the capacity for personal growth, having everyday living conditions as far as possible like those of the general community and promoting physical and social integration in the life of the community. All of the new laws emphasized that when decisions are made on behalf of people with a disability they must be decisions that are the least restrictive of that person's freedom of decision and action. Included in these laws were provisions to establish the Office of the Public Advocate. This agency operates independently of government with responsibility to promote the interests of people with disabilities and to protect them from abuse, exploitation and neglect.

The observations in this chapter are drawn from the work of the Office of the Public Advocate in providing advocacy services for individuals and groups, advocacy in relation to systemic issues and in providing services as the guardian of last resort.[1]

A report to the Premier of Victoria in 1977 described large institutions as characterised by overcrowding, understaffing and under financing. They have effectively segregated retarded people, isolating them from contact with the general community and providing them with a deficient living environment...' (A Report of the Victorian Committee on Mental Retardation 1977, 113). These isolated and routinized environments were highly protective and restrictive with limited opportunities for self-expression or exploration of individual potential or character. For an overwhelming proportion of those people who moved from such institutions into the community, or who subsequently have never moved into an institution at all, the outcomes have been beneficial. That fact must be emphasized lest it be overlooked in the observations that follow.

We concede that the nature of the Public Advocate's role as an advocate or guardian of last resort means that the Office sees some of the most intractable problems and the most disturbing instances of exploitation and abuse. Nevertheless, the reality is that for some people with an intellectual disability the process of deinstitutionalization has led to new forms of care and management that are institutional in nature.

Case study: Jason

Jason is a 25-year-old man with a moderate intellectual disability. During his lifetime he has lived with his family, in an institution and also in a community residential unit run by the Department of Human Services with other residents with intellectual disabilities. At times he has worked in supervised employment settings.

Over the past ten years Jason has been the perpetrator of abuse involving young children on a number of occasions, the most recent of which resulted in a 12-month prison sentence. As his time for release drew near, a number of professionals were concerned that he would re-offend. These concerns were expressed in terms of the potential dangers that this would present to younger members of the community (on whom he seemed to focus his sexual attention) and also with reference to the risk that Jason would return to prison, any reconnection with the criminal justice system not being perceived as in Jason's best interests. Health professionals who knew Jason believed that he could receive treatment, over an extended period of time, to assist in his development of more appropriate sexual behaviour and that, eventually, this might enable him to live within the community with appropriate supports.

As no legal mechanisms existed to compel Jason to receive the long-term treatment he required,[2] the civil mechanism of guardianship was used to detain him in a secure treatment facility. The Victorian Civil and Administrative Tribunal appointed a guardian as it found that Jason was a person with a disability, that his disability impacted on his reasonable decision-making and that there were current decisions that needed to be made. The tribunal appointed the Public Advocate as guardian with power to make health-care and accommodation decisions. The guardian made an accommodation decision that Jason should reside in a secure treatment facility in Melbourne.[3] Jason has remained in that facility for over two years. In effect, therefore, the guardian's decision has civilly detained Jason for an indefinite period, ultimately dependent on his treatment progress. While this decision may be in Jason's best interests, his liberties are curtailed as a consequence. In earlier years Jason, particularly after his offending behaviour became known, would almost certainly have been held in an institution. The same was probably true for many others who were like Jason, even if their offending behaviour was not as serious. Now, although they may not be truly integrated into the community, they are free to move about in it and do, as a result of their behaviour, come into contact with the criminal justice system. A lack of the capacity to control one's actions or appreciate the effect that they have on others or to recognize that those actions are wrong can result in serious offending behaviour. Alternatively, the behaviour may be more of a nuisance value but can lead to the accumulation of thousands of dollars of unpaid fines or repeated court appearances that exhaust the ingenuity or capacity of the law for diversion. For many the freedom of being in the community has allowed the freedom to make the same mistakes as others: mistakes such as the misuse of drugs and alcohol. Combined with their disability, this has made them particularly at risk of arrest, of conviction and of failing to meet the conditions of community corrections orders and therefore at risk of imprisonment. Increasingly, the lower criminal courts report higher proportions of accused persons with an intellectual disability. In turn, the prisons are housing people with an intellectual disability at a much higher proportion than they represent in the population as a whole. Thus, for too many the move from institutions into the community has meant a move to another form of institution far more restrictive of their freedom, namely prison.

In the case of Jason and others like him, the disability services system has sought to prevent this from happening but it has done so in a way that, from his point of view, may seem to be little different from a prison. Arguably, the imposition of a programme of cognitive behaviour therapy is of benefit to him and, if successful, will provide him with the opportunity to move back into some form of community living. The options for accommodating people with a disability who are assessed as presenting a risk of serious harm to others are very limited. In some cases it can result in living alone in a suburban house: alone, that is, except for the two carers who keep watch 24 hours a day. For some it is sharing with some three or four others a house that is kept securely locked. In each of these cases the imposition of the accommodation regime amounts to civil detention. Added to these options is the use, in some situations, of what amounts to chemical incarceration; that is, the use of drugs not with the primary purpose of treating an illness but to restrain and to modify behaviour.

The reality is that in Victoria many decisions are made that restrict fundamental freedoms of movement or decision-making, without any legal framework for doing so. Only under mental health laws is there a provision for involuntary detention. The law relating to the provision of services to someone with an intellectual disability is voluntary in its nature. That is to say, people can only be provided with services if they agree to request them. Advocates in the 1980s sought, quite properly, to separate mental illness from intellectual disability both legislatively and administratively. One reason for the difference in approaches is that mental illness is perceived as being treatable: mental disorders can be remedied or at least the symptoms can be ameliorated. It is therefore possible in mental health law to set up a tension between the right to individual autonomy on the one hand and the right to treatment on the other. Such is not the case with intellectual disability which cannot be treated in the way that a mental illness can.

The consequence is that the prospect of community living is replaced with a form of civil detention without a legal framework and without any guarantee that the decisions made are those that give effect to the option that is the least restrictive of an individual's freedom. Nor is there any guarantee that the decision is made in the best interests of the individual rather than the interests of others or to cover up the failings in the service system. Finally, and important, there is no system of independent, external review of the decisions to protect the rights and interests of those with the disability.

The appointment of a guardian in Jason's case and in a small number of others where the risk is not to the person with a disability but to other members of the community is quite inappropriate even though it does provide him with some degree of protection. A guardian, charged with the responsibility of acting in a person's best interests, is more properly appointed when someone needs to be protected from harming themselves or to be protected from exploitation, abuse or neglect.[4]

Jason's story illustrates one of the ways in which moving out of an institution into the community can mean moving into another form of institution. Both feature decisions imposed upon him without transparent, reviewable processes and without proper accountability for the decision-makers. For some, like Jason, these restrictive outcomes are the consequence of the complexity of their needs and the inadequacy of the system in responding. Mental illness disproportionately affects those with an intellectual disability and substance abuse is too often an additional factor. The service system, established to assist those with a disability or an illness or an addiction, struggles to cope with a dual or multi-diagnosis or disability. It is when the system fails to provide solutions that meet such complex needs that prisons replace institutions and other forms of restrictive living environments replace community living.

Case study: Maria

Maria is in her mid-forties and has spent a large part of her life in institutions. She has a moderate intellectual disability. In recent years, Maria has been relocated to a community residential unit in a suburban locality of Melbourne. She shares this house with four other women and care staff.

A number of Maria's co-residents is inclined to wander. In response to this risk, the community residential unit is secure, with staff responsible for ensuring that the facility is locked and unlocked as needed. It is not possible for residents to enter or leave the facility without staff to facilitate their access, thus creating an atmosphere of inflexibility and regimentation. While Maria herself is not at risk of wandering, she must experience a more confined living environment as a consequence of the needs of her co-residents. Her personal liberty is significantly restricted.

Essentially, this case study illustrates the failure of the accommodation system to meet Maria's particular needs. She is exposed to the deprivations imposed by the lowest common denominator approach. This approach means that, because Maria resides in a community residential unit with other women whose wandering habits require their liberty to be curtailed, Maria's freedoms are also restricted as she is captured by the restrictive response to the group as a whole. A more appropriate response would witness a careful grouping of residents according to their abilities and safety needs.

Perhaps what most characterizes Maria's institutionalization is its subtlety. To the casual observer, she lives in a group home located within the community. Yet she is kept in, locked in, to accommodate the needs of her co-residents, while the community is symbolically kept out. This mirrors the classic institutional context despite the fact that it is dressed in the clothing of integration within the local setting.

Of particular note is the fact that Maria has no choice in relation to those with whom she lives, a right or decision which most of us simply take for granted. She also has limited opportunities to negotiate the rules of the household, including those related to entry, exit and access regimes. The issue of how people with intellectual disabilities can effectively participate in decision-making that fundamentally affects their lives is complex. It remains an area which would clearly benefit from further exploration.

Maria may also be disadvantaged in her environment by the disproportionate time which is required of staff members in the community residential unit to attend to the more complex needs of the other residents whose behaviour puts them at greater risk. In turn, this may have implications for Maria's own development and her ability to reach her fullest potential. This can be characterized, to some extent, as a restriction on her liberty to grow. In addition, the skills and capacities of staff may also be affected by the extent of use of casual staff in the unit who are less familiar with Maria's needs. Staff, whose work practices mirror those of large institutions to the extent that large congregate-care centres were their training grounds, may need to learn new ways of caring for clients, if the individual liberties of these clients are not to be undermined.

Maria's situation could be improved by an increased focus on her needs, specifically a more appropriate accommodation option. This may have resource implications and would certainly require more vigorous advocacy in which Maria's own needs and interests would be more clearly represented, and responded to, in the decision-making process.

The case study illustrates the invisibility of Maria due, in part, to the systemic failure to adequately meet her housing and support needs. In so doing, this reminds us of the decades of invisibility to which people with intellectual disabilities have been exposed, mirroring, once again and ironically, the institutional context. Maria therefore experiences a form of subtle neglect which leads to her experience of a new form of institutionalization, at once both insidious and perhaps less open to scrutiny as it is overtly accepted as appropriate and integrated community living.

Conclusion

Emerging from the two stories are those factors that can contribute to situations in the community that create new forms of institutions. Deficient or inadequate legal frameworks for compulsory care and treatment for those with an intellectual disability lead to decisions that are not transparent, nor subject to appeal, and which do not ensure that the decision-makers are held to account for ensuring that solutions which are least restrictive of individual freedoms are found. Inadequacies in service infrastructure that lead to a failure to meet a diversity of needs with varying complexities, inadequate resourcing and a lack of commitment to trialling a variety of accommodation options, and the use of inappropriately trained and resourced staff, can all contribute to the replication in a community setting of those deficiencies that characterized the old institutions.

There remains, too, a need for improved mechanisms for the involvement of people with intellectual disabilities in decision-making which affects them: exploring and taking into account their wishes and with mechanisms to monitor their concerns and needs.

Overwhelmingly, deinstitutionalization has brought about positive improvements in the lives of many, but there are those for whom the change has been little more than a change of address.

Notes

1 Under Victorian law a guardian is appointed by a separate tribunal if it is satisfied that a person has a disability and is unable because of the disability to make reasonable judge-

ments, and that there is a need to appoint a guardian. The powers of a guardian cover some or all lifestyle decisions: accommodation, access to other people or to services, health care and employment. They do not include power over financial matters.

2 Under the Mental Health Act 1986, an involuntary patient can be treated without his or her consent provided that he or she meets the legislative requirements for involuntary status. Treatment can occur in an institution or in the community, under a 'community treatment order'. However, there is no equivalent regime in Victoria for the compulsory care and treatment of those with an intellectual disability. Generally, the receipt of services by a person with an intellectual disability requires that person to be an eligible client and to actively agree to receive such services. In complex cases this is often difficult to achieve.

3 Essentially, the decisions of guardians are not reviewable. What is reviewable is the guardianship order itself.

4 However, it is noted that the Victorian Law Reform Commission released a report in November 2003 entitled *People with Intellectual Disabilities at Risk: A Legal Framework for Compulsory Care.* This report recommended legislation to provide an appropriate legal framework for making such decisions that has at its core the promotion of benefits to the individual. The government is currently considering that report.

References

Guardianship and Administration Act 1986 (Victoria).

Intellectually Disabled Persons' Services Act 1986 (Victoria).

Mental Health Act 1986 (Victoria).

Victorian Committee on Mental Retardation (1977) *Report to the Premier of Victoria.* Melbourne: Victorian Government Printer.

Victorian Law Reform Commission (2003) *People with Intellectual Disabilities at Risk: A Legal Framework for Compulsory Care. Report.* Melbourne: Victorian Government Printer.

20

Returning to One's Roots

Haki Titori's Story

Patricia O'Brien, New Zealand

Haki Titori is a man who is a descendent of Ngapuhi, which indicates he came from the far north of New Zealand. As a teenager with a disability who was blind, he had some behavioural problems and his family agreed to place him in an institution. I first met Haki when he was nearly 50. He had lived in an institution for close on 30 years. I was involved in helping him leave the institution to live in the community.

The move was not easy for Haki. He disliked his new house and indicated this to staff by not letting them near him. He often spent whole days making loud noises. The neighbours began to complain. The staff tried lots of ways to support Haki. But in the end he returned to the institution. I drove him back and can still remember how sad I was as I left him. Haki, however, seemed pleased to be back in a familiar place even if the chair he was sitting on was broken.

The next move out of the institution for Haki was much more successful. He moved into a house that was run for Maori men by Maori staff. Here he was able to get in touch with his heritage. Staff spoke Te Reo, his Maori language, and cooked Maori food for him and took him to Maori activities, such as weaving and concert groups. Haki was surrounded by members of his *whanau*, which is a Maori term for family. With the staff who have become part of his *whanau*, Haki is leading a much happier life. Recently, after 40 years, he was reunited with his brothers. Staff from the service found his family and invited them to come down from the far north to Auckland for Haki's sixtieth birthday. Although Haki is blind and does not speak, the staff believed that he did recognize his family. He sat beside them and listened to their voices in a manner that indicated that he knew who they were.

Haki is a respected member of the *whanau* that now surrounds him within the service: Te Roopu Taurima O Manukau. Within this service he has been assisted to regain his well-being both physically and spiritually. Haki has regained his spirit and is acknowledged as an elder of the community in which he has found his place. Community living for Haki has meant that he now belongs.

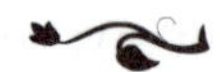

Patricia writes: The story that follows demonstrates the bicultural nature of Aotearoa New Zealand, which has a population of four million people, 12 to 15 per cent of whom are Maori. Underpinning life in New Zealand is a partnership between Maori and the European population (*pakeha*). This partnership is enshrined in the Treaty of Waitangi, which was signed by Maori chiefs and representatives of the British Crown in 1840. The story tells what life is like for a Maori man who is living in a service developed by Maori for Maori. A separate service within the context of biculturalism has enabled this man to find his roots after a lifetime of institutionalization.

Haki's story

It was a holiday weekend and, as I drove through the suburbs to where Haki (Hacki) had lived in a regular house on a regular street for the last six weeks, I was sad. On a day when most people were relaxing and enjoying an extra day's break,

I was driving to pick up a 50-year-old Maori man and return him to the institution where he had lived for the past 30 years. This was so different to the many times that I had driven people away from the institution to a new address in the community with hope and anticipation of a changed life. Haki's life had changed. He had moved into a house on a suburban street with four other people. His arrival and stay had not been smooth, resulting in neighbours taking up a street petition to have him removed.

In response to the community reaction, the transition team that I worked with had increased support hours for Haki and had worked more intensely with staff, but the opposition from the neighbours was not to be assuaged. Of the 61 people with intellectual disabilities who had left the institution and gained a new address, Haki became one of only two people to be returned. I led the transition team and have often reflected upon what else could have been done to overcome what became a period of reinstitutionalization for Haki. The answer lies in how his story unfolds.

Basically, Haki was returned to the institution because of constant loud wailing that the neighbourhood was not able to tolerate. Certainly, staff members were also challenged by his incontinence, as well as his aggressive reaction to being physically encouraged to participate in self-help and recreational activities. Given time, these issues would have been overcome, but time was not on Haki's side, but on that of the agitated local community.

I have a vivid memory of his return to the institution, his near-empty ward and his joy at walking out into a concrete-paved area and sitting in a broken-down chair, his chair of many years. With the sun shining, complacency came over him. This was his home and, regardless of its degradation, it was where he wanted to be. As I said goodbye I did have a sense that he did not share my sadness. He had stopped wailing.

It was almost ten years before I saw Haki again. I was at the opening of Te Roopu Taurima O Manakau, a service which

> has the responsibility of ensuring that the provision of services for people with disabilities meets their needs in a holistic way, representing individual dignity and encompassing all dimensions of Tikanga, as well as the four cornerstones of health. (Christensen 1997a, p.162)

As a member of the service, Haki was seated with the elders at the opening ceremony. The contrast with the time I left him back at the institution was dramatic. Here was a man who was composed, emanating a sense of belonging. It occurred to me that all those years ago, if his heritage had been planned for in the transfer, he might have found his place in the community earlier.

Following Haki's return to the institution, he was transferred to another community-based service but this service had a cultural aspect to its provision. He lived in a house for Maori people, managed and staffed by Maori. This part of the service eventually broke away from the mainstream service to become Te Roopu Taurima O Manukau Trust. On a recent visit to where Haki is living supported by this service, I sat with him and with his staff and reminisced about his life since leaving the institution. Although Haki does not make conversation, he sat at the table for a large part of the *korero* (talk, conversation). Staff approved having their reflections tape-recorded, on the understanding that the story would be returned to them for verification before it was published. Throughout the story the word 'staff' will, in keeping with *tikanga* (Maori principles, customs and procedures), be used interchangeably with *whanau* (family).

As I approached the house to meet with Haki and his *whanau*, my emotions ran high to see the quality of Haki's home. It was a large house with an attractive external appearance, the type of house that is often built for families on a section of several acres. As I entered the house, I saw that the contrast to his previous life was stark. The earlier images of people like Haki sitting in a day room, their lives wasted for up to 30 or more years, often dressed only in surgical gowns, waiting for meals to arrive, was now replaced by Haki and flatmates sitting on comfortable sofas, enjoying CDs, interacting with *whanau* or watching television. Here there was no furniture with foam coming through the chair covers and no area bare of any personalized mementoes. Photos of trips and activities were evident in the house. This was a house where the people who were non-verbal were much respected. This was a house where the four cornerstones of Maori health were holistically pursued for all four men that lived there. Interaction between the men and their *whanau* aimed to ensure their:

- *te taha wairua* – spiritual well-being
- *te taha hinmengaro* – mental well-being
- *te taha tinan* – physical well-being
- *te taha whanau* – family well-being (Christensen 1997a).

The dignity with which Haki, a 60-year-old man, now lived his life was exemplified by how his goals were recorded. Unlike the clinical hospital files, he now had his own leather-bound and zipped diary. Within the A4-sized diary Haki's life, since being part of Te Roopu Taurima O Manukau, was profiled. It was a living document, indicating how his current goals were progressing, as well as including two daily diary entries, throughout the current year. Accompanying his diary was his photograph album. It was obvious from these documents that being in this service was enabling him to experience the culture that he was born to. His *whanau* was committed to ensuring that his culture, denied by years of institutionalization, was given back to him.

As I sat at the dining-room table with Haki and the staff who were playing a significant part in his life, I came to learn that his living situation revolved around *tikanga* (Maori principles, customs and procedures), including his food. The following comment from one of the staff encapsulates this:

> You wouldn't get that in any other service...it is important that they have their type of inheritance integrated into their lives. It is about valuing them, for who they are as individuals. I'm not trying to say that other services don't do that but I think Maori just does it differently. We respect a person for who they are, where they come from and have an understanding of what this means and its importance.

For Haki, in living outside the institution, his inheritance had become central to his life. Its impact has ranged from simple pleasures to events of major significance. Whatever the complexity, all activities were planned to be part of a holistic approach to the healing of his *wairu*, his Maori spirit.

Simple pleasures were described as listening to music, having a boil-up, drinking the soup of the boil-up, eating bread and hearing his language being spoken in the home, as well as being shown respect by being referred to as *koru*, a term of endearment for an older person. Such routine activities have been underpinned by what was the most significant event of all, which was Haki's being reunited with his family after 40 years. This must be directly attributed to his placement in a Maori service. At the time of his first leaving the hospital, staff members were unsuccessful in tracing his family, but his *whanau* at Te Roopu Taurima O Manakau was successful.

> We went up north and found the family and invited them to his sixtieth birthday. So they came down here, the two brothers and sister-in-law, and it was as though he knew. [Uncharacteristically] he sat so quietly... I think there had to be some link, he was familiar with them being right next to him. He didn't scream.

Forty or more years had passed since the family had seen their brother. This could have happened earlier if, at the time of his leaving the hospital, the transition team, of which I was a member, had worked in partnership with Maori. Thirteen years later a transition team would never have been envisaged without such membership.

In terms of healing, being reunited with his *whanau* would have provided Haki with 'the opportunity to participate in the life [he] was born to' (Christensen 1997b, p.58). It enabled his *whanau* also to share their early memories of Haki. A most poignant memory was 'how their mum used to have Haki out on the boat with them fishing. Although he was blind he used to still have his own fishing line.' This memory was significant for the staff, as one of the activities that they had identified as giving Haki pleasure was fishing.

The meeting with the family was made more touching by the fact that soon after Haki's birthday, one of his brothers died. His *whanau* within Te Roopu Taurima are continuing to keep the contact alive with a trip planned up north for Haki to stay on his local *marae* (a traditional place for Maori people to gather).

Following deinstitutionalization, stories of community living often focus on increased activity and strengthened friendship networks (O'Brien, Thesing and Capie 1999). For Haki, the journey since leaving the institution has been different, focusing more on being reunited with the community of his birth – his *whakapapa* and *whanau.* Over time, staff members have worked to re-establish these links, enabling Haki to experience *te wheua* (land), *te reo* (language), *te ao turoa* (environment) and *whanaugatanga* (extended family). As such, his membership of Te Roopu Taurima has worked to establish his personal worth. In keeping with the premise of Royal (1988), his healing from years of institutionalization has come about from staff working with him to answer the questions of 'Who am I? Where do I belong? Where am I from?'

Life since moving away from the congregate care within the institution has enabled Haki to learn 'self-help-type things, hand-washing, putting his own clothes on without him standing there waiting for someone to do everything for him'. Haki is seen by staff as a person who despite earlier deprivation can still learn. The commitment of staff to ensuring Haki's ongoing development was expressed as follows:

> We find that even with the age he is and the experiences he's had, he can still learn and it's quite empowering when you realize you can still teach him.

Teaching goals for Haki were often not new but assisted him to unlearn the survival skills of institutionalization. In relation to eating independently, one staff member reflected:

> When I first came to work with him, going back to his eating, there was always a big rush and it was like [he was thinking] 'someone is going to take this from me. I need to eat it as quickly as possible', and it took some time, but eventually, to a verbal prompt, he would slow down and put his utensil down and swallow and have a break, and then would pick it up and start again. Whereas earlier it was just non-stop until his plate was finished.

In setting goals, the staff were realistic, indicating that they needed to be achieved 'within a certain time frame' if Haki was not to become agitated. This was connected to their belief 'that he obviously hadn't had the best of life and it had taken him a long time to trust'. Te Whetumarama (the name of his house) had provided Haki with a safe environment. His security was evidenced by his decrease in anti-social behaviour. Ear slapping and loud repetitive vocal noises, as well as spontaneous urinating, had decreased and trust was shown now in the way that Haki would allow staff to guide him to places. Previously he 'didn't like being touched'. Put succinctly by staff: 'He really has changed...his life is a good life now...he's come a long way.'

At 60, and ten years on from leaving the institution, Haki's life was continuing to evolve and the dreams for his future expressed by his *whanau* would see him sharing with:

> Another person of his age, possibly with the same fragilities, but they would have one-on-one staffing. In the meantime as long as he's got his rocking chair and a regular cup of tea and he's warm and cosy, he feels very comfortable within himself.

As I left Haki, he had moved from the dining-room table to a small sitting room especially set up for him to listen to his music while relaxing in a lazy-boy armchair. He looked very comfortable within himself. Here was a solitary man who enjoyed his own company. Community living for him meant security. His needs were being met in a holistic way, with his individual dignity being respected and who he was as a man being understood. His *whanau* ensured that his life now was relevant to his heritage.

As I said goodbye to Haki I was no longer saddened by his circumstances as I had been all those many years ago when I drove him back to the institution. Living within a service that had a commitment to *tikanga* had made all the difference for Haki.

Rapua Te Ara Tika Mou Ake

Search for the path that is right for you.

Epilogue

After Haki's story had been written, Patricia O'Brien received a letter from Lorraine Bailey who directs the service where Haki lived. The letter is below.

Kia Ora Tricia

I have sad news of Haki, that I thought I should pass on to you. On 12 August 2003, he passed away due to a blood clot on his brain. He died very suddenly at home, while soaking in a warm bath. He always enjoyed his evening bath, and staff couldn't understand when he made strange gurgling sounds, followed quickly by unconsciousness.

Haki lay in state in our *Wharehui*, E Tipu E Rea, on Gadsby Road, for two days and one night. This allowed the Mokopuna and Kaimahi throughout the service to pay their respects to him. His *Kuia* and *Kaumatua* were there as well, and accompanied him back to his *Marae* in Rawhiti, Bay of Islands. Members of our staff and management team with Mokopuna from Te Whetumarama, also travelled North to be there for his funeral service and burial. At our *Wharehui*, Te Roopu Taurima O Manukau Service had a formal *Kai Hakari* to farewell him from Auckland. His *whanau* were so pleased with the *Awhi* and *Tautoko* shown to their *whanau* member.

His funeral service was conducted by Bishop Ben Tahara, his uncle, and he was interred on the top of a hill overlooking both sides of the Bay of Islands. He lies with his parents and grandparents, as well as other *whanau*. His brother who had died previously lies just along from him.

So he did a complete return journey back to his roots, and his beloved ocean where he fished with his mother 50 plus years ago. He really was the respected *Koro* of our service, and particularly the Kaimahi who supported him in his everyday life.

Moe Mai E Koro, Moe Mai.

I do hope you go ahead with publication, and I will give consent for the story to be told.

Noreira, nga mihi aroha kia koe Tricia me to hoa Tane, Ray.

Nga mihi atu nei.

Lorraine Bailey

References

Christensen, L. (1997a) 'Te pumautanga: A perspective on the development of human services.' In P. O'Brien and R. Murray (eds) *Human Services: Towards Partnership and Support.* Palmerston North: Dunmore Press.

Christensen, L. (1997b) 'A reflection.' In P. O'Brien and R. Murray (eds) *Human Services: Towards Partnership and Support.* Palmerston North: Dunmore Press.

O'Brien, P., Thesing, A. and Capie, A. (1999) *Living in the Community for People with a Long History of Institutional Care.* Auckland: Auckland College of Education.

Royal, T. (1988) 'A discussion paper.' In N. Harrison (ed.) *Racial and Ethnic Issues in New Zealand Polytechnics.* Wellington: Department of Health.

21

Becoming Contractual

The Development of Contracts and Social Care Markets in England

Paul Cambridge, UK

As people with intellectual disabilities moved out of institutions to live in the community, different ways were found to provide them with services. In the past, most people with disabilities in England received services from the government. Now things are different, as services are provided by many different agencies and people in many different ways. Some of these include contracts for particular services and the use of care managers who help people find services and work with agencies to make sure that services are co-ordinated.

These ways of providing services can work well in that individual needs are taken into account and people with intellectual disabilities have more choices and power over the kinds of services they receive. So Rachel, who did not have help with communication when she lived in an institution, received good communication support and a wheelchair once she had moved out, and so was able to lead an active life in the community. However, there are also problems with having contracts for services. People with intellectual disabilities may not be asked what they think about the contracts for their services. Sometimes agencies are paid money and make agreements which are not in the best interests of people with intellectual disabilities. It is important that services are paid for and provided in a way that respects the right of people with disabilities to have a say about their own lives and to get the things they want in the community. One of the best ways to do this is to give people money so that they can arrange their services either themselves or with the help of an advocate.

Introduction

As a child I was fascinated by a neo-Gothic building on a hill overlooking the A2 London-to-Dover road. I later discovered that it was one of the largest 'mental handicap' hospitals in southern England (see Korman and Glennerster 1990 for an account of its closure). When I was working in Somerset there was a huge effort to close the three mental handicap hospitals in the county, which together accommodated over 400 people. My anti-institutional views were strengthened by the images I witnessed when later visiting residents in the hospitals included in the 'Care in the Community' programme (Knapp *et al.* 1992). Some had been workhouses, such as the Nora Fry hospital in Somerset. Here I spoke to an elderly woman who had been admitted 60 years earlier because she had an illegitimate baby. I walked corridors of over a mile long and across caged iron walkways in St Lawrence's hospital south of London, looking for staff or patients. I stumbled on a party, held by staff, from which patients were excluded. Other hospitals comprised 'villas' in the grounds. Whatever they looked like, these places reflected total institutions (Goffman 1961, Foucault 1977).

My uncle Arthur had a severe learning disability caused by Down's syndrome and was unable to communicate verbally, feed, wash, shave or toilet himself. After living at home with my grandparents in a small village on the North Downs and later with my family, he was moved to Leybourne Grange Hospital and, when it eventually closed, back to the community through a home-care placement. Shortly after being in the second placement he was admitted to hospital seriously ill. We were told by social services that he had developed a serious allergic reaction to drugs. However, the consultant considered that Arthur's injuries were consistent with scalding in a very hot bath. Social services refused to arrange allergy tests and when the carer was asked what medication was involved and the name of the GP, the story was changed. It was then alleged that he had eaten a poisonous plant in the carer's garden. At this point I contacted the police. Arthur died in hospital two weeks later after being in continuous pain. At the inquest the pathologist described him as a 'low grade Mongol'. The coroner recorded an open verdict. I witnessed my mother's anguish.

My research and personal experience therefore informed me about the links between deinstitutionalization and the development of contractualism. In many ways what happened to Arthur was a consequence of the failure of contractualism as well as community care. I had expressed concern at the time of his placement that his care management was too closely allied to his placement, compromising independence and advocacy. Effectively, contractualism was about getting him out of hospital and into a private and largely unregulated care setting. Here, the competence needed for his care was not only absent but also invisible to others, outside of independent scrutiny of the quality of his support.

Defining contractualism

The notion of using contracts as a device to manage community and social care is highly contentious. Views tend to be polarized according to political belief and values. This was reflected in the way social policy in England developed in relation to community care and the social-care market. The 1990 community-care reforms (Department of Health 1989) separated purchasing from providing, and introduced contracts as a device to manage care markets under a Thatcherite Conservative administration. Conversely, New Labour intervened to manage and regulate the social-care market and encouraged agencies to work together in partnership, reducing reliance on contractual relationships.

Contractualism in social care is therefore a very complex subject which draws on theory and practice in economics, consumerism and organizational change. For the purpose of this chapter, however, I will define contractualism as the formal relationships which were developed between agencies following the separation of purchasing from providing after the 1990 community-care reforms in England. These were centred on the device of the contract and operated in the context of a social-care market. Contracts in social care represent legal agreements between the purchaser and provider of services, and specify what services are to be provided. Depending on the types of contracts, they may also specify in relation to service provision: how, where, in what ways and who for. Block contracts, for example, cover a whole service provided for a number of people, while individual contracts cover services for one person. Contracts vary in their robustness and capacity to specify things such as the quality of services, how service users are supported in their daily lives and how performance is reviewed.

Contractualism in England developed in parallel with the transfer of people with intellectual disabilities from institutions to community care. To some extent this chapter also seeks to illustrate the relationship between these two movements. The complexities of contractualism in a social-care market, such as that operating in England, suggest the need for an analysis which examines contractual relationships at a number of key levels, namely between agencies, between individuals working or operating in care markets, and in relation to the role people with intellectual disabilities themselves can play.

The big players in contractualism: a game played between agencies

Care markets and contracts are known to operate imperfectly. The distortions and anomalies in services generated by social care markets in England have been well documented (Forder, Knapp and Wistow 1996; Wistow *et al.* 1994), including those in intellectual disability (Cambridge 1999a; Cambridge and Brown 1997). Because of their limits, such markets are termed quasi-markets (Le Grand and Bartlett 1993). Indeed, they have developed within various constraints, including internal markets in health, incremental contracting out of social care in local government and more competitive provider markets in the voluntary and private sectors (Butler 1992; Wistow *et al.* 1994).

In the mid-1980s, the Audit Commission (1986) recommended that local governments should be made responsible for the long-term care of 'mentally and physically handicapped people in the community' and that the resources necessary to do this should be transferred from the NHS (National Health Service). The importance of developing unambiguous lead responsibilities and funding for an emerging mixed economy of care was thus recognized. The trend towards markets culminated in the separation of purchasing from providing and overt contractualism in *Caring for People* (Department of Health 1989).

Social services departments in local government became lead agencies for purchasing community care. They were also responsible for providing care management and assessment, including services for people with intellectual disabilities. Community-care plans were required in their localities, and consumer involvement and individual choice were promoted as objectives within a consumerist model.

However, there was no evidence that markets and contracts would work in social care. People with intellectual disabilities are not powerful consumers who can take their custom elsewhere and were invariably not party to contractual agreements about their services (Cambridge and Brown 1997). They effectively became commodities traded between agencies through block contracts and cost-led purchasing. The primary players were health- and social-care agencies, building on the relationships developed from joint planning and joint finance (Cambridge 1999a; Waddington 1995) and also the imperative to move people out of hospitals, which were NHS provided, to community care, which was largely provided by social services. Whilst this was generally undertaken in planned ways, social-care markets often took over in determining what happened to people with intellectual disabilities living in the community.

Public assets, and those previously held collectively by people with intellectual disabilities, were largely transferred to the control of barely accountable agencies, often removed from public scrutiny and service-user control. There was a parallel disinvestment in human capital, through the fragmentation and de-unionization of the workforce, and the declining pay and conditions of employment (Cambridge and Brown 1997). In a five-year follow-up study of deinstitutionalization (Cambridge, Hayes and Knapp 1994), we witnessed the separation of purchasing from providing services and the emergence of the opportunities and risks that contractualism brings (Cambridge *et al.* 1994).

Opportunities included more efficient division of responsibilities between agencies; the potential to devolve authority and budgets closer to service users through care managers; incentives to develop cost-effective services; greater consultation and co-operation and the development of partnerships between agencies and the articulation of responsibilities and expectations through contracts. However, risks were also apparent. These included service fragmentation and loss of direction; wasteful duplication and rivalry; diminishing public accountability; cost-led purchasing; increasing inequities between different service users and authorities; high levels of transactional costs; confrontation between commissioners and providers of services; short-termism and the exclusion of service users.

The 12-year follow-up (Cambridge *et al.* 2002) revealed that few of the opportunities flagged in the earlier research had been realized while many of the risks had materialized.

With New Labour came a stream of policy initiatives designed to focus on co-operation, partnership working, performance management and consultation (Department of Health 1998a, 1998b, 1999). This was effectively market management expressed through best value, care standards and inspection. This new cycle of regulation came barely ten years after the largely failed experiment of deregulation through care markets and contracts, which it was assumed would deliver competition, economy, quality, choice and user involvement. Indeed, special policy instruments such as person-centred planning, direct payments and advocacy needed to be introduced or promoted to encourage user involvement and choice in the newly regulated care markets (Department of Health 2001).

The individual players in contractualism: co-ordinating services in care markets

The second level at which contractualism operates is in the relationships between care managers, service users and carers. Care management has been used as a device to co-ordinate services across a care market, working from assessment and individual service planning, and in many cases using individual contracts for services, although its implementation has been hugely variable (Cambridge 1999b). Care management therefore has the potential to play a direct role in contractualism through micro-purchasing, but this raises critical challenges for care managers and service users.

To act as purchasers with or for people with intellectual disabilities, care managers need access to good information on service costs and quality, linked to information systems on individual service use and the costs of individual service packages. Cost information is generally held by commissioners at the aggregate or macro-levels at which commissioners generally contract for services, so it is often difficult for care managers to purchase one-off services. The other general difficulty with contractualism is that there is rarely information on individual outcomes and quality. The information which is easiest to collect is not necessarily that which is most helpful for purchasing good quality and safe services for people with intellectual disabilities.

Brokerage and direct payments to individuals represent more overtly consumerist approaches to contractualism for people with disabilities, although these are only now beginning to be more widely used and tested (Dook, Honess and Senker 1997; Dowson 1995; Values into Action 1994) as part of new government policies in relation to people with intellectual disabilities (Department of Health 2001; Holman and Collins 1997).

Checks and balances are particularly important in these approaches to help ensure that people with intellectual disabilities are not exploited by carers or workers. Person-centred planning is proving an effective way to help ensure that people with intellectual disabilities are not excluded from decision-making, which will be especially important as brokerage services become more widespread.

If this trend is to develop, it is important that care managers be able to develop a relationship with the people with intellectual disabilities whom they serve, so that professional advocacy can ensure that users of services actually get the services they need and want, and that accountability for public funds is maintained. However, for this to happen there will need to be limited caseloads for care managers, few cost constraints in relation to service purchasing and clear divisions between those who commission services and those who provide them (Cambridge 1999b). Self-advocacy groups also offer a good way for people with intellectual disabilities to be represented in contractual relationships, such as those developed through direct payments.

Partnership boards were recently established between the new primary-care trusts, which were health agencies responsible for services for people with intellectual disabilities, and social services departments. This provided opportunities for service users to be represented at the highest levels of service organization. For example, in recent work in Kensington and Chelsea I have seen user and self-advocacy groups represented on the bodies which commission services for people with intellectual disabilities and a quality network of service users undertaking inspections of the services provided. This contrasts hugely with the relative lack of participation and choice which people with intellectual disabilities were given during deinstitutionalization and the early days of social-care markets.

The user-consumer: people with intellectual disabilities themselves

In theory, contractualism was meant to lead to more individualized services and greater consumer choice. As the social-care market was a natural experiment in England, as it varies so much between localities and as it had become increasingly managed, it is of course very difficult to make definitive judgements about user benefits. Moreover, other policy interventions have to be taken into account, such as the introduction of person-centred planning and direct payments. In relation to the shift to deinstitutionalization, key messages from longitudinal research on outcomes and costs for people with intellectual disabilities have revealed that the greater individualization, which has been made possible for some services by using a more contractual approach, has been important in improving the quality of their lives (Cambridge *et al.* 2002; Forrester-Jones *et al.* 2002). The story of one woman I worked with illustrates this.

When Rachel first moved out of hospital she pulled herself around the house on the floor. Her verbalization, facial expressions and signing were not readily understood. She was labelled as having challenging behaviour, biting her hands and lips and screaming. She did not engage with support staff and was unable to participate in everyday activities or decision-making. However, thanks to the more individualized services provided by contractual arrangements between agencies alongside the changing values of individual community care, Rachel gained greater control of her physical and social environment, made far more choices, expressed her preferences and achieved her goals. A new communication system together with her motorized chair enabled her to become more independent, visiting her local pub or the jazz club and ordering her own taxi via a connection to the telephone system.

The things that service users value in their lives in this time of more individualized services reflect the sort of things we all value. They include privacy, choice, friendliness of neighbours and the convenience of local amenities, as well as the comfort and quality of the accommodation. Yet these are the very aspects of quality of life which prove difficult to specify and monitor through contracts. Similarly, the most frequently mentioned problems occurring within the social milieu include bullying, the living regime and the physical aspects of the accommodation, along with personal feelings of loneliness and boredom. A substantial minority of service users was not happy with the degree of privacy and choice afforded, and only half had positive relationships with neighbours (Forrester-Jones *et al.* 2002 and in press).

Although service users are recognized in research (Cambridge and Forrester-Jones 2003; Emerson and Hatton 1994; Nocon and Qureshi 1996), less progress has been made in including them in contractual relationships or care management, although mechanisms such as individual service specifications could be used (Cambridge 1999b). However, with the intellectual disability White Paper, *Valuing People*, placing emphasis on person-centred planning more centrally in relation to contractualism, and direct payments (Department of Health 2001), new approaches outside care management have emerged. Experience to date remains mixed, although distinct advantages and disadvantages are evident with direct payments (Carmichael and Brown 2002). Advantages of this approach for service users include more choice, control and flexibility. Disadvantages include complexity for the service user and the restraint of innovation in more complex service packages.

Conclusion

Contractualism is slowly being introduced across most developed social-care economies, like it or not. There remain alternatives to relationships developed through contract or the exchange of resources. In Sweden, for example, services are still publicly led and provided, and remain highly individualized and localized. The potential also exists to explore the collective ownership of assets by people with intellectual disabilities themselves.

The greatest challenge is undoubtedly to make contractualism, at whatever level and form, work for people with intellectual disabilities, and there are examples from commissioning and direct payments where this does happen. It is often forgotten that contractualism brings additional transactional costs and we need to be confident that the benefits and achievements outweigh these. We also need to ensure that if we have social-care markets, then they are well managed and inspected to the benefit of service users and public finance.

Contractualism, in whatever form, needs to be guided by a shared commitment to deinstitutionalization, desegregation and individualization – with service purchasing grounded in 'Ordinary Life' models (King's Fund 1980), 'The Five Accomplishments' (O'Brien 1987) and anti-oppressive practice (Williams, Keating and Nadirshaw 2002).

A number of recent abuse scandals in England underline the capacity of community-care services to develop abusive cultures (Cambridge 1999c; Longcare 1998; Macintyre 1999). The task of contractualism is to ensure that this does not happen; that Rachel's story is repeated and Arthur's story is not.

References

Audit Commission (1986) *Making a Reality of Community Care.* London: HMSO.

Butler, J. (1992) *Patients, Policies and Politics.* Buckingham: Open University Press.

Cambridge, P. (1999a) 'More than just a quick fix? The potential of joint commissioning services for people with learning disabilities.' *Research, Policy and Planning 1*, 2, 12–22.

Cambridge, P. (1999b) 'Building care management competence in services for people with learning disabilities.' *British Journal of Social Work 29*, 393–415.

Cambridge, P. (1999c) 'The first hit: A case study of the physical abuse of people with learning disabilities and challenging behaviours in a residential service.' *Disability and Society 1*, 3, 285–308.

Cambridge, P. and Brown, H. (1997) 'Making the market work for people with learning disabilities: An argument for principled contracting.' *Critical Social Policy 51*, 27–52.

Cambridge, P., Carpenter, J., Beecham, J., Hallam, A., Knapp, M., Forrester-Jones, R. and Tate, A. (2002) 'Trends: Twelve years on – the long-term outcomes and costs of de-institutionalisation and community care for people with learning disabilities.' *Tizard Learning Disability Review 7*, 3.

Cambridge, P. and Forrester-Jones, R. (2003) 'Using individualised communication for interviewing people with intellectual disability: A case study of user centred research.' *Journal of Intellectual and Developmental Disability 28*, 1, 5–23.

Cambridge, P., Hayes, L. and Knapp, M. (1994) *Care in the Community: Five Years On.* Aldershot: Ashgate.

Carmichael, A. and Brown, L. (2002) 'The future challenge of direct payments.' *Disability and Society 1*, 7, 797–808.

Department of Health (1989) *Caring for People: Community Care in the Next Decade and Beyond.* London: HMSO.

Department of Health (1998a) *Partnership in Action.* London: HMSO.

Department of Health (1998b) *Modernising Social Services.* London: HMSO.

Department of Health (1999) *A New Approach to Social Services Performance.* London: HMSO.

Department of Health (2001) *Valuing People: A New Strategy for Learning Disability for the 21st Century.* London: HMSO.

Dook, J., Honess, J. and Senker, J. (1997) *Making Changes: Service Brokerage in Southwark.* London: Choice Press.

Dowson, S. (1995) 'Service brokerage: The alternative to care management?' *Values into Action Newsletter No. 81.* London: Values into Action.

Emerson, E. and Hatton, C. (1994) *Moving Out: Relocation from Hospital to Community.* Manchester: HARC, University of Manchester.

Forder, J., Knapp, M. and Wistow, G. (1996) 'Competition in the mixed economy of care.' *Journal of Social Policy 25*, 2, 201–221.

Forrester-Jones, R., Cambridge, P., Carpenter, J., Tate, A., Beecham, J., Hallam, A., Knapp, M., Coolen-Schrijner, P. and Wooffe, D. (in press) 'The social networks of people with learning disabilities living in the community twelve years on.' *Journal of Applied Research in Intellectual Disabilities.*

Forrester-Jones, R., Carpenter, J., Cambridge, P., Tate, A., Hallam, A., Knapp, M. and Beecham, J. (2002) 'The quality of life of people twelve years after resettlement from long stay hospitals: Users' views on their living environment, daily activities and future aspirations.' *Disability and Society 17*, 7, 741–758.

Foucault, M. (1977) *Discipline and Punishment.* London: Allen Lane.

Goffman, E. (1961) *Asylums.* New York: Anchor.

Holman, A. and Collins, J. (1997) *Funding Freedom: A Guide to Direct Payments for People with Learning Disabilities.* London: Values into Action.

King's Fund (1980) *An Ordinary Life.* Project Paper No. 24. London: King's Fund Centre.

Knapp, M., Cambridge, P., Thomason, C., Beecham, J., Allen, C. and Darton, R. (1992) *Care in the Community: Challenge and Demonstration.* Aldershot: Ashgate.

Korman, N. and Glennerster, H. (1990) *Hospital Closure.* Milton Keynes: Open University Press.

Le Grand, J. and Bartlett, W. (1993) 'The theory of quasi-markets.' In J. Le Grand and W. Bartlett (eds) *Quasi-markets and Social Policy.* London: Macmillan.

Longcare (1998) *Independent Longcare Inquiry.* Buckingham: Buckinghamshire County Council.

Macintyre, D. (1999) *Macintyre Undercover.* BBC1 TV documentary, 16 November.

Nocon, A. and Qureshi, H. (1996) *Outcomes of Community Care for Users and Carers.* Buckingham: Open University Press.

O'Brien, J. (1987) 'A guide to lifestyle planning.' In B. Willcox and G. Bellamy (eds) *The Activities Catalogue.* Baltimore, MD: Paul H. Brookes.

Values into Action (1994) 'Choice and no choice.' *Values into Action Newsletter No. 7.* London: Values into Action.

Waddington, P. (1995) 'Joint commissioning of services for people with learning disabilities: Review of the principles and the practice.' *British Journal of Learning Disabilities 23*, 2–10.

Williams, J., Keating, F. and Nadirshaw, Z. (2002) 'All different, all equal: Understanding and developing anti-oppressive practice.' In S. Carnaby (ed.) *Learning Disability Today.* Brighton: Pavilion.

Wistow, G., Knapp, M., Hardy, B. and Allen, C. (1994) *Social Care in a Mixed Economy.* Buckingham: Open University Press.

22

The Dignity of Risk

My Son's Home and Adult Life

Dóra S. Bjarnason, Iceland

My son Benedikt is 23 years old. He is like other young men in that he loves life, girls, music, dancing, basketball, swimming and travel. He goes to work and spends his time with friends and family. He is unusual in that he was born with significant impairments and needs help at all times.

Benedikt has always been in regular schools and had many friends in grammar school. Many of them are still his friends. I asked his friends to help us plan Benedikt's future as an adult. We played the game: 'What would Benedikt say if he could talk?' Five things stood out: he would want to go abroad to study or work, have his own home, continue with his music, have a job and spend time with friends. Based on this, Benedikt's future was planned.

Benedikt went to Denmark for a year of study and when he came home he moved into his new home in a lovely apartment close to downtown Reykjavík. Benedikt needs a lot of support to live in his home. Young people who live with him provide this support. Some of his friends also make sure things are working well for him, as well as family members.

It took a long time to find a job for Benedikt but he now works part time in a large church in downtown Reykjavík selling admission to the church tower. Benedikt also takes music lessons and goes to concerts of the Icelandic Symphony Orchestra.

Benedikt seems secure in his new life. Anyone who meets him can see he is a very happy young man. He is not able to say what he wants but he can show his preferences through body language, facial expressions and pointing. His way of expressing himself is respected and he has many opportunities to take part in the same activities as other young people his age. Benedikt has a good life but he is very dependent on the people around him.

Benedikt's story

My son Benedikt Hákon Bjarnason is in many ways a typical young man. He loves life, girls, music, dancing, basketball, swimming and travel. He goes to work and spends his spare time at home with other young people, or out with his friends or family. He is unusual, however, in that he was born with significant impairments which have resulted in a number of labels, such as intellectual disability, epilepsy, spasticity and more. He needs intimate personal help at all times. He also needs people who can help him express his needs, wishes and longings, and who can stand up for his rights.

Benedikt is 23 years old and was born in Reykjavík, Iceland. He belongs to the first 'inclusion generation' of disabled Icelanders. With the supports made available by the welfare state to disabled children, teenagers and young adults, Benedikt has led his life as a fully included, active member of his society. He went to a regular preschool, an ordinary compulsory school and a regular technical high school, and he went abroad to study at a youth college in Denmark. In the summers, Benedikt went to ordinary summer programmes and summer camps for kids and, like most of his generation of Icelandic youth, he had a few summer jobs in his teens tending to parks and delivering newspapers. As a boy he made a number of friends amongst his classmates who came to our house to play with

Benedikt one day a week, most weeks, for the best part of his ten-year compulsory schooling. Benedikt was also invited to some of their homes for birthdays or other special events.

Many of these childhood friends are still part of his life, but the tasks and challenges of young adulthood have temporarily separated many of them and spread them between universities in Iceland and abroad, on the labour market or on exploratory journeys to see the world. Benedikt has also travelled extensively. Being a university professor, I have had the opportunity to travel and live in other countries during my sabbatical leaves. Benedikt has always been with me. As a result, he has lived and gone to school in six countries on three different continents and travelled to many more countries during his life. (More about Benedikt and his life can be found in Bjarnason 2003.)

Planning for the future

As Benedikt grew up I worried what would become of him as an adult. He has always been included in all aspects of community life and I could not imagine him in some form of group facility for disabled people or a segregated day programme. As his schooling came to an end, the problem posed itself with increasing urgency: how can a young man like Benedikt lead a full active life within society; enjoy privacy, choice and autonomy; have friends and support himself on a disability pension? What kind of lifestyle would he choose? His friends and I played the game: 'What would Benedikt say if he could talk?' We drew up a long list of things he might want to try. Five things stood out: he would want to go abroad to study or work, get a home of his own, continue with his music, get a job and go out with friends from time to time. On the basis of this I drew up a plan for Benedikt's future.

The process of moving into an adult life started in the autumn of 2000 when Benedikt went abroad to Denmark for one year of study at Egmont College with his friend Fridrik Rafn Gudmundsson. Fridrik attended the same college and took on being Benedikt's helper during the year. A sabbatical leave enabled me also to spend the academic year 2000–2001 in Denmark. This was the first time my son had moved away from home and I felt it was safer to be in the same country. However, I was in Copenhagen, which is in a different part of Denmark, so we only saw each other irregularly on weekends and school holidays.

Before leaving for our year-long stay in Denmark we had, with the help of some good professionals, made a plan for Benedikt's interdependent living in a home of his own and had signed the agreement for its implementation upon his return from Denmark in 2001.

A home with support

The negotiations with representatives of the Reykjavík social services office and the State-run Department of Disabled People's Affairs in Reykjavík started in 1998 and the ideas evolved over a two-year period. These negotiations centred on how we could create a home for Benedikt. The project was called 'Home with Support' (Bjarnason 1999). I worked on this in the dual role of a parent and of a university researcher and teacher of disability studies. Benedikt's home provides an example of how it is possible to reach the goals of a regular life in the community as defined by the Icelandic disability legislation (Act on the Affairs of Disabled People 1992). The project was developed as an experiment in co-operation with officials from the disability service sector and the municipal social services in Reykjavík. Benedikt's 'Home with Support' was inspired by a similar home developed by two American professors, Dianne L. Ferguson and Phil M. Ferguson, who are also parents of a young man with significant impairments, but I adapted it to fit Icelandic culture and welfare provisions.

Benedikt's support needs are extensive and complex. If he were to move into a group home, it would cost the State the salary of three to four workers, depending on the size of his private space and the service needs of the other residents. In addition, the State would pay towards day services or a sheltered workshop and for transport. When all the costs of group-home placement and related services (as they are defined by Icelandic welfare legislation and social policy practice) were added up, it became clear that a person could be provided with a more appropriate and inclusive lifestyle for less of the taxpayers' money. The authorities agreed that some of this money would go directly to Benedikt in order for him to be able to pay his helpers and cover the cost of special services.

I carved out a support plan, intended to work even without my presence, that would enable Benedikt to explore his adult lifestyle choices. The organizational structure is as follows:

- *The board.* This is a board of management, consisting of seven of his childhood friends and schoolmates from compulsory school, a man with a good understanding of finances, a human rights lawyer and his mother. The board meets *ad hoc,* and at least once a year. Its responsibility is to step in at times of need and secure the continuation and safety of Benedikt's home, possessions and lifestyle.
- *The personal agent.* This is a hired professional who manages Benedikt's helpers, solves practical problems, suggests new things and helps make sure that Benedikt's lifestyle and quality of life remain as

appropriate for his age and interests as possible. The agent's contract states that he will, if at all possible, only quit this job after hiring and training his successor.

- *The helpers.* Benedikt has three helpers on a daily basis. Currently, these are young people his own age who share his home and take turns in supporting Benedikt in his daily life. Benedikt has certain routines; apart from that his helpers use their own imaginations. They take Benedikt along to activities that they all like, and bring their own friends and interests into their joint home.

In the spring of 2001 I found a spacious apartment well suited for Benedikt's needs. Five of his Danish schoolmates, who came to Iceland in the spring term in search of adventure, moved into the apartment temporarily and paid the rent by painting it. The apartment is well located in a house with five other apartments and in a good neighbourhood. It is in a popular part of Reykjavík, within walking distance of the city centre where young people gather, near a public recreation area, shops and one of the town's most popular outdoor swimming pools. Benedikt and three helpers – Fridrik and two Danish school friends, Ali and Helle – moved into the apartment in late June 2001.

The apartment has become a lovely home. Benedikt's schoolmates from Denmark had more than paid for their keep. The sitting rooms and bedrooms were beautifully painted in pastel-green colours. Parquet has been laid on all the floors and a new bathroom and kitchen have been installed. I moved every piece of furniture I could do without into the apartment and bought some more second hand. We hung various paintings Benedikt had acquired and photographs from his life. With a piano, a television and a music centre in the sitting room, and curtains for the windows, there didn't seem to be much wanting.

The moment I had longed for and prepared for more carefully than anything I had ever done in my life had finally arrived. Benedikt had left home. It had been a carefully crafted and planned project but it was also very emotional. At the time I wrote in my diary:

> My darling son, it is high summer but autumn is round the corner. You are twenty-one years of age, and full of light and happiness. Ali and his fiancée are visiting, they have brought the Egmont spirit of friendship with them. I am fifty-five today. I am happy that I have managed to support you, but only the future can tell what awaits us. I miss your daily company more than words can express, but rejoice all the more over the time we spend together. It is lovely being invited to your home for supper, or visiting Granny, going

> for a drive in the country or to a concert. I often ask myself whether I have done the right thing and whether I would do the same again, given another chance. There are no satisfactory answers to these questions. I shall simply have to have faith in your good fortune and in kind people, and hope that you will not suffer for the fact that I made your life into an experiment. When I was told that you were so disabled that you might as well be left to 'lie in bed and grow' I gave you a promise that I would make your life as rich as possible, that it would be of use and happiness to you as well as other people. You yourself have fulfilled this promise I gave you as a baby in my arms. Life is a risky business, but it is also beautiful. (From Dóra S. Bjarnason's diary)

Benedikt's adult life

The years that have followed have brought many new experiences for Benedikt and his friends. A few weeks after he moved in, we invited some of his old childhood schoolmates for a visit and I detected a trace of envy over his home. They also celebrate his new life and some of them are on the board for Benedikt's new home.

With the board and other arrangements in place, I felt we had created the safety net which is necessary for the future if Benedikt is to be able to live in his own home. With all of this in place, officials from the local Department of Disabled People's Affairs and from Reykjavík's social services office came to Benedikt's home for lunch one day where we formally signed the contract for an experimental project called 'Home with Support', initially valid for two years. The contract commits the two agencies to paying Benedikt the cost of the wages for his three helpers.

Benedikt lives on his disability pension which just about covers his daily needs. A small allowance from his parents makes some luxuries possible. House bills are split four ways and each person pays a small rent that goes towards paying the mortgage. The four young people who share the home have a joint budget for food and they share the housework. Running the car is my responsibility and, though it is mainly used by Benedikt and his helpers, we share ownership of it.

Benedikt's life has followed a similar course to that of his non-impaired peers. For a while work was the only area where he was held back. It took much effort to find work for him after he returned from Denmark. Every employer we spoke to received us kindly but every place seemed to be in the process of reorganization and the personnel manager was unable to meet Benedikt, let alone find out about his abilities and what he and his helpers would be able to contribute.

Finally, Benedikt was given the opportunity to make a contribution, thanks to one of my colleagues who is a chaplain at Hallgrímskirkja, a large church in downtown Reykjavík. Benedikt works there two mornings a week as a volunteer, selling admission to the church tower to tourists. This is a great workplace for Benedikt; the tourists like meeting him and his helpers take the money while Benedikt hands over the tickets. The church's organ is the biggest and best in Iceland, and Benedikt enjoys listening to the organist when he practises.

Benedikt has been to a full season of concerts of the Icelandic Symphony Orchestra and attended the Kópavogur School of Music where he studied electronic composition, which he thoroughly enjoyed. One of his compositions was performed in the students' spring concert in one of Iceland's finest concert halls.

The helpers have been wonderful and Benedikt loves being surrounded by people his own age, going places and doing things with them. The only complaint is that these young people do not remain for more than a year as his helpers. This means that Benedikt's quality of life depends on our continuing success in finding new helpers and teaching them how to help him. One of the most difficult aspects is teaching these young people to help him to be himself, rather than a pocket version of themselves. I, on the other hand, have to learn to draw a clearer line between myself as Benedikt's mother and him and his helpers. So far, most of the young people have become my friends but this may not remain so; a woman in her fifties has a different outlook on life from youngsters in their twenties. The personal agent is very important in helping me and Benedikt keep a mother–son relationship and freeing me from being the manager of his home.

There are a few drawbacks to the way Benedikt's new life is organized. One is the high staff turnover. His helpers are close to him in age. These are young people who wish to continue with their studies and they usually only stay for 8–12 months. This cannot be helped if he is to live with young people. We have built in a mechanism which ensures that old helpers train the new ones. Another drawback is that Benedikt's old friends often need to speak with relative strangers when visiting him. I fear this may deter some of them from visiting. Finally, there is Benedikt's vulnerability and the fact that his quality of life rests on trust in the people who work for him. These are risks and drawbacks he must live with but they are possibly not different to those in the average group home.

Benedikt seems secure in who he is. Anyone who meets him can see that he is a very happy young man. He gets ample opportunity to take part in life and various activities and events he chooses with help from his peers, helpers, personal agent and family. He may not be able to voice his preferences but he receives support to access age-appropriate cultural events, and his ability to show his preferences via body language, facial expressions and pointing is respected.

Benedikt is now 23 and, though I have Power of Attorney, he is legally of age. He exercises his citizenship rights and voted at the last local elections. He lives a good life in peace with his family and his neighbours. His adulthood, however, is different from that of most other adults. He cannot look after himself unaided. He is an adult with the help of the people who surround him and who speak for him. I have chosen risk above safety. I hope I have made the right choices. Benedikt's existence and quality of life are precarious. They depend on his beiðng surrounded by enough people who care about him and look after his interests as an adult.

References

Bjarnason, D.S. (1999) 'Heima er best: jónusta viþ fatlað folk sem býr á eigin heimili og þarf mikinn stuðning' ('Home sweet home: Services for disabled people who live in their own homes and have high support needs'). *Uppeldi og menntun* ('Upbringing and education') *8*, 55–69.

Bjarnason, D.S. (2003) *School Inclusion in Iceland: The Cloak of Invisibility.* New York: NOVA Science Publishers.

Lög um málefni fatlaðra nr. 59/1992 (Act on the Affairs of Disabled People, no. 59/1992).

23

Out of the Institution Trap

John O'Brien, USA

The institution is a trap for people. Just getting out of the institution doesn't mean getting out of the trap. People with disabilities can be kept apart from other people, treated as if they were less valuable than other people and controlled by staff even in an ordinary house.

It does not have to be this way. People with disabilities and their allies have learned how to assist people to make choices, make valuable contributions and participate in community life. To learn how to do these things people have to get out of the ways of being with each other and thinking about each other that keep them in the institution trap.

We have read about Tom Allen in each part of this book. Many bad things were done to Tom in the big and small institutions he lived in. He fought back and took as much freedom as he could, no matter how hard the institution tried to own his life. Tom's story shows us ten ways to fight the institution trap.

- Reach out and make friends.
- Remember the people who have loved you. Remember their love even if they have also let you down or hurt you.

- You can find spaces to be free if you learn all about how the institution controls people.
- Find safe ways to use your voice. Don't give up when others don't listen.
- Be a decision-maker.
- Learn to do whatever you can for yourself, even if it is hard and takes a long time.
- Make a positive difference to other people with disabilities.
- Don't think like the institution. The institution wins when you give up and believe that you are no more than the institution thinks you are.
- Tell and retell your own life story to anyone you can trust to listen.
- Keep your dream alive and guard it from people who try to kill it.

> Lobster pots are designed to catch lobsters. A man entering a man-sized lobster pot would become suspicious of the narrowing tunnel, he would shrink from the drop at the end; and if he fell in, he would recognize the entrance as a possible exit and climb out again.
>
> A trap is a trap only for creatures which cannot solve the problems that it sets. Man-traps are dangerous only in relation to the limitations on what men can see and value and do. A trap is a function of the nature of the trapped. (Vickers 1970, p.15)

The institution trap is crafty

As lobster pots are to lobsters, so institutions for people with intellectual disabilities are to us: deeply dangerous and revealing. Energized by our collective uneasiness with imperfection, dependence and mortality, institutions trap us. We mindlessly impose segregation and supervision on people who require accommodation and assistance due to impairments in learning, communicating, or moving –

treating them as if they were devalued or dangerous or disgusting to 'Others' (Nussbaum 2004). That we apply the cosmetics of cure, care or choice only makes the trap more alluring, keeping ordinary members of the public at a distance, detachedly admiring the work of those so busy with assessments and activities and treatments that the entangling mesh escapes notice.

The institution trap is protean. When it can no longer ensnare large numbers in a collection of buildings crowned by a water tower, it shifts its shape and assumes the disguise of an ordinary-looking house. Maria (Chapter 19) makes her life with four other women whose tendency to wander is managed by staff who lock the doors rather than imagining and practising a life with their charges that might be more engaging than playing endless games of containment and escape. Such imagination and practice would be informed by positive approaches to dealing with troubling behaviour (Lovett 1996), but such interventions cannot work apart from an organizational culture that encourages staff to recognize and delight in a sense of common humanity. Such a sense allows staff to discard the mask of impersonal overseer. Apparently caught along with staff lacking this vital imagination and skill, Maria remains suspended in the institution trap, her situation recounted here only as a commentary on the reproduction of nineteenth-century patterns in twenty-first-century places.

For those concerned more with offering people a good life than with supervising their maladaptive behaviours, it is possible to backtrack from even a big mistake and find a way to slip through the institution trap. Haki (Chapter 20) finds his familiar broken chair in an institution ward superior to being placed in a five-person group home. He reverses this decision when fellow Maori invite him to take a seat among the elders. Themselves taking a stand for the value of their culture by creating a Maori service, these staff join Haki in escaping the institution trap. They respect the dignity of his age, reunite him with his extended family and live in ways intended to heal his Maori spirit. This second chance is the product of personal relationships between people who value their shared identity as Maori, an organization dedicated to asserting the specific contribution that Maori culture can make in a service world dominated by European values, and a political climate shaped by the assertion of Maori rights and disability rights.

The institution trap is systemic. Arthur (Chapter 21) died painfully and unnecessarily from scalding. His fatal injury was not sustained in a large public institution but in a community home, whose operators ineptly tried to cover up the cause of death, maybe to protect their trading position. The state pathologist and the coroner assigned no fault in the death of this person, described in their record as a 'low grade Mongol'. Arthur's move from the institution into a lethally incompetent situation lacked the safeguard of any authoritative way to review the facility's competencies and comforts from Arthur's perspective. Instead, his placement was driven by a political priority that ignored his interests: the creation of a contract-based market in community care serviced by private entrepreneurs and fed by the closure of publicly operated institutions. People can have more security, even within the constraints of a system designed to offer contractors advantageous business conditions (Cambridge 1999), but such safeguards take thoughtful design and painstaking implementation.

The institution trap is crafty. Some people with mild intellectual impairments, like Claes (Chapter 18), have escaped disability-service-enforced segregation, but not a form of social isolation that greatly increases the risk of addiction and anti-social behaviour. In an earlier generation, Claes might have found himself preventatively detained, living as a 'working boy' in an institution for the mentally retarded. Today the prison system does the work of institutionalization as Claes joins too many other unsupported, isolated people with mild intellectual disabilities in jail. As those who created Meeting Place No. 10 know, it is possible to generate positive ways to confront social isolation and devaluation, but this effort has come too late for Claes. Other people, like Jason (Chapter 19), are entangled in a net woven of ineffective responses to what could be a compulsion to abuse children. The accumulation of difficulties and support failures led the intellectual disabilities service system to export him: first into the prison system and then into indefinite detention in a secure mental-health facility under the authority of a public guardian. It is not necessary that the institution trap claim Jason. There are forms of assistance emerging that protect other citizens while assisting a person to live a life that makes sense. However, even limited success requires a depth of knowledge and wisdom that can only be acquired by service workers who are willing to recognize humanity in people who do truly scary and sometimes bad things, and who are willing to learn how to mindfully surround opportunities for growth with protection (O'Brien *et al.* 2003).

Resisting the institution trap from inside

Fans of *Star Trek: The Next Generation* have met The Borg, a cybernetic life-form whose mission is to improve the quality of life for all those they meet by assimilating them, discarding their cultures and identities and amalgamating them into an efficient machine-like collective. Their monolithic spacecraft harnesses great technological power to enforce their greeting to strangers: 'You will be assimilated'. To those who object to assimilation, they matter-of-factly respond: 'Resistance is futile'. Of course, in *Star Trek*, as in life, the interesting stories unfold through the actions of those who believe that resistance is possible, even if risky and often less than fully successful. The institution trap is implacable and its impersonal technologies can strip away people's humanity but, like The Borg, its power multiplies when people buy the story that resistance is futile.

Learning to see resistance

Fixating on wounds caused by the cogs of the institution trap can obscure the agency and creativity of those caught in its gears. It can be tempting to cast institution inmates as simply passive victims, waiting, as inert as Snow White, for a rescuer to appear. Alternatives and advocacy are surely necessary to get people out of institutions, but a more nuanced view is available to those who practise seeing the ways institutionalized people carve out moments of meaning and freedom. Understanding how to see and encourage these capacities for resistance is critical to moving beyond the institution trap.

Bob Williams (2004) – poet, alternative communication user, disabled policy analyst and activist, and Clinton Administration US Deputy Assistant Secretary for Disability, Aging and Long Term Care Policy – demonstrates the appreciative, open and unhurried gaze necessary to recognize 'the subtleties of the moment' that reveal how two institutionalized people 'knowing that they're all they have...learn to make do'.

Dick and Jane

They've shared the same mat since they were children,
lately though the staff has been setting them down
so that they're facing in opposite directions of one another,
probably to avoid any funny stuff.

It doesn't matter that much though;
they'll nestle together no matter what,
knowing that they're all they have,
they learn to make do.

Her body is that of a child
though her face is taking on the features of a beautiful young woman;
looking into her hazel eyes, I'm almost mesmerized by their sparkle,
it took me a while to figure out the score.

Finding pleasure in giving her lover a back rub
with spasmodic strokes of her arm, she massages the small of his back;
smiling, he responds in kind by running his whiskers through her toes,
she gives out a slight laugh;
they move an inch or two closer to each other
hoping that the staff doesn't pick up on the subtleties of the moment;
they don't of course. (Williams 2004)

Remembering the danger

Though resistance is possible, it is often dangerous. Tom Allen (Chapter 17) was 'put in a corner, facing the wall, for hours on end simply for talking out of line'. Other inmates saw him and learned. The institution trap can close very tightly indeed around those who resist openly. As Bob Williams shows (2004), violence against resisters can be cloaked as therapy. Others saw what happened to Johnny and learned.

The Marathon Man

Johnny ran
that was his problem,
he was what the staff called a runner
logical since he ran whenever he could

one minute
they thought they had him
three ways to sunday
tied to the bedpost
with someone else's soiled sheets;

then they'd no sooner turn around
and he'd be up to his harry houdini
routine all over again.

even the aides admitted he was pretty
smart for being a retard;
all the rest of them would sit and rock.

but not Johnny
he'd jump up
dart this way and that.

then the next thing you know
he'd find an open door
or leap through a window

and he'd be clocking the mile
on the institution's main drag
at three-point-ninety-two
like the long distant runner he longed to be.

they tried vinegar spray,
four-point restraints,
even leaden shoes.

nothing slowed his free stride
until they placed electrodes on his hide
and shocked him.

shocked him silly.

now he's on the back ward
rocking to and fro
to and fro
to and fro… (Williams 2004)

Learning to make do

Tom Allen learned to make do in very constrained circumstances. By passing on the gift of Tom's autobiography (Chapters 1, 7, 12 and 17), the editors of this book honour one of the projects that brought meaning to his life: teaching lessons in how people should not be treated and how those subjected to such treatment can assert their freedom despite an impoverished, isolated, controlling environment. They also provide a catalogue of the ways the institution trap works and how to resist it.

Being caught in the institution trap brought Tom many troubles. The Epilogue says that he suffered much more than he wrote, but he wrote about troubles enough. The next few paragraphs detail the workings of the institution trap on Tom. Abstracting these insults to Tom's humanity yields a list so cold as to be false to Tom's mostly gentle, hopeful way of telling his story. In his telling, the warmth of his generosity and hopefulness balances the coldness of the treatment that tempts him to bitter anger and despair. However, the chill of enumerating some of what Tom endured gives proper proportion to the acts of resistance Tom authored.

Tom was taken away from his family twice by a system with no capacity to support his family to raise him. The doctor in the institution specialized for his care sent Tom home to die when he was six years old.

Tom recounts four years of troubles after readmission at age 16. His desire to make some of his own decisions kept him in trouble with staff. He was not allowed to bring his belongings from home (and did not have any personal belongings for another 32 years). He wore hospital clothes. 'No school. No work. No physical therapy. No speech therapy. No nothing' (Chapter 1). Throughout his long stay in this facility, dental work meant extractions but no dentures, a practice that made it harder and harder for him to eat as the years went by. Though he had occasional letters, he had no visitors for five years. His anger at abandonment grew and he began to question whether even God was still with him. 'My desperation was so deep it is hard to describe' (Chapter 1).

Anger and desperation led him into bigger trouble with staff, which resulted in demotion to a poorer ward to live with more severely disabled people. Tom shifted his survival strategy and turned what was intended as punishment into roles meaningful to him, which he continued to play for many of the next 37 years. Moving to an institution closer to his family led to the loss of his role as a helper. 'I just sat around all day and was terribly bored' (Chapter 1).

At age 69, Tom had his own room for the first time in his life – this lasted for about a month before he moved to another institution in order to improve his chances of finally moving into a group home. In this facility, for the first time in his life, he lived on a ward and had meals at a table that included women. While this facility offered some new opportunities, it also posed new threats. Tom was repeatedly victimized by other residents and lived in fear that he could not defend himself and that staff would not protect him. His glasses were broken repeatedly. Money and clothing were stolen from him. Food was taken from him and thrown at him. He withdrew into his room for self-protection. But, for Tom, there was something worse than physical victimization and restrictions on his movements, which he presents in his court petition for an injunction to provide him with a community placement.

> I have been frequently disappointed by the state's broken promise to find a home in the community for me. This has been the worst indignity and disappointment I have suffered.
>
> ...I am often depressed; I worry about whether I will ever live in the community before I die. (Tom Allen's affidavit, Chapter 7)

After two and a half years of hard work, Tom moved into a community residence with three other people, returning to the institution to spend his days for two years and then, after 'retirement', sitting in the residence with nothing to do. The stress of living with constant fear that his nightmare would come true and he would be returned to the institution aggravated his stomach problems.

Despite a more home-like, physically safe setting, there was the disappointment of another failure to meet Tom's modest expectations.

> Moving into the community did not bring me the freedom I had dreamed about. I was still quite isolated. All the lists I made about all the things I wanted to do seem to have disappeared...
>
> I can have my say and express my wishes but the staff make the rules for the most part and make the decisions... As soon as I have learned to like the staff, chances are they will quit... Some of the staff do not like helping me eat. They think it takes too long and I can feel they don't want to be bothered.
>
> I was getting very tired and disappointed. My health was failing. I was losing weight and what was worse, I was losing hope. I did not even want to talk. I wanted to die. (Tom Allen, Chapter 12)

Tom summed up much of his life experience in a speech against institutions. 'I felt like I was in prison being punished like a criminal and all I had was a disability' (Chapter 17). Being taken from and feeling abandoned by his family, both in infancy and in adolescence, are wounds that could shadow a whole life. Most of the insults to Tom's humanity were day-to-day, year-in year-out experiences that grind away at human dignity and vitality: nothing meaningful to do, being ignored or offhandedly punished for voicing his perceptions and desires, surviving on a meagre diet with limited medical care in a barren environment, waiting for one of the parade of arrangers and co-ordinators sent by the State to make good on its promises.

Tom's strategies for resistance allowed him to make do with whatever his environment made available to him. When there was more to work with – as in his time as a helper in H-Building and in the last ten years of his life – he was better able to resist the institution trap. In my reading, Tom created at least ten ways to hold on to his own life within the institution trap.

The institution isolates you and subordinates your relationships to its human-management interests; *reach out and make friends.* Make friends among the people you live with and especially with those members of staff who are free enough to rise above the social norms that cast staff as impersonal overseers. Keep making friends even though people keep leaving. Whenever there is a chance, make friends from outside, as Tom did when he was finally able to attend church. Tom involved his friends in his life projects, drawing them closer to him. When rendered idle by lack of opportunities, he began to dictate his autobiography to helpful staff, whom he was concerned to protect, even to the extent of keeping their names out of his autobiography's acknowledgements. Late in his life, Tom's friends helped him make major changes in the way his assistance was organized and delivered, so that he could have greater control of his daytime.

The institution discourages involvement with your family; make whatever contacts you have as nice for your family members as possible and *take nourishment from the memory of those who have loved you.* Tom's remembering positive times with his mother and grandmother soothed him and inspired his dream of once again being part of a loving family. Tom is generous in his account of his father and his brothers and sisters. He welcomed their occasional visits while acknowledging that he felt that they had mostly abandoned him.

The institution controls the smallest details of your daily life; *read the environment to find cracks* in the regime. Tom found and occupied niches for himself even in difficult environments like the back wards. When he lived on a ward that didn't allow its residents outside, he noticed that smokers could leave and tried smoking.

The institution wants to silence you; *find safe ways to use your voice and don't give up just because others don't act on your messages.* When, at age 69, he encountered a resident government, he became its vice-president. When given the invitation to list his preferred activities, he did so. When he met a lawyer at work on closing the institution, he became a plaintiff. When people were organizing to close institutions, he spoke out at their meetings and in hearings. When he lost hope and the will to live, he responded to his friends' invitation and joined in planning and implementing his personalized retirement programme with great pleasure.

The institution makes decisions for you to protect you from risks; *see yourself as a decision-maker and take risks to improve the chances of getting what you want,* even when the only decisions you can make concern your own attitude toward things. After being moved as a punishment, Tom decided that his survival depended on not only following the rules but helping staff out and getting them to like him. Tom moved from setting to setting to get closer to his dream. By the time of his kidney failure, he had enough support and clarity of purpose to refuse the dialysis that would have put him back in a nursing home. The hospital stays during which he had to make these decisions were less stressful for him because, thanks to his friends, he was never alone.

The institution makes you dependent; *learn to do what you can for yourself.* Tom organized other residents to help him to eat so that he did not have to depend on hurried staff. He learned to push himself in his own wheelchair. He found ways to do tasks the staff saw as helpful.

The institution has low expectations of you; *create ways to contribute.* For years Tom organized the work of other inmates to ensure that people in his building with more substantial disabilities were cared for. He worked hard to finish his autobiography before he died so that others could learn from it.

The institution gets inside your head and the heads of some of the people you care about; *challenge the depression, inaction and fear that comes from thinking like the institution.* Tom noticed the error of believing that the State's refusal to assist him to move out of the institution was because he wasn't working hard enough to better himself. Instead of trying to earn his way out by changing himself, he looked for opportunities and help to move toward his goal. When Tom's closest brother said he didn't want Tom to move from the institution, he listened but took his own course.

The institution wants to own you and your past; *tell and retell your own story* to yourself and anyone you can trust to listen.

The institution wants to own your future; *keep your dream alive and guard it from people who would try to kill it.* Dreams matter as guides and as a source of strength whether or not they actually come true.

> I wanted to be part of the world and wanted to leave the institution. I dreamed about the things I would do when I left. I dreamed of having a wife and children, I really wanted to have a family; my own family like my wife and children. A happy family like we had been before my mother died. What I wanted most of all was to have a wife; a woman that I loved and who loved me back. This dream is what kept me going. It kept me alive. During times of despair I turned to it and it comforted me and gave me strength. I have held on to this dream all my life and never stopped hoping it would come true. (Tom Allen, Chapter 17)

Better living conditions and more professionals do not necessarily add up to more freedom, as Tom discovered when he moved to the group home. Greater freedom to live among friends as a contributing citizen is what makes for a good life, and freedom is what the institution trap squeezes out of people's lives. Moving on from institutions calls for learning how to dissolve the institution trap.

Dissolving the institution trap

Tom spent his whole life seeking the assistance that he required to pursue his interests and contribute to others' well-being. In his last years, he and his friends pushed back the walls of the institution trap far enough to allow Tom personalized support during 'day-programme hours' (six hours a day on weekdays). Lisa, an assistant Tom chose, listened to what he wanted to do and helped him do it. His desires were simple: sharing a familiar routine that begins with the daily paper; calling and visiting family and friends; going to familiar places in his community – the library, the swimming pool, the Farmers' Market, shopping for foods he prefers and occasionally for clothing, sometimes visiting a bakery with particularly good chocolate éclairs; advocating for institution closure; working to find a family interested in sharing their lives and offering Tom a real home; and, sometimes, breaking routine with a camping trip, a visit to the state fair or a trip to a family reunion or to visit a relative who lives far away. What made these 30 hours a week life transforming for Tom is that he had freedom-in-relationship with Lisa. Tom planned with Lisa to set his schedule and select his activities, and worked out what he wanted from a particular activity or encounter. Then Lisa assisted him to deal in positive ways with the way his mobility and communication impairments might interfere with his purpose (see Traustadóttir 1991). Though time ran out before Tom was able to further escape the institution trap by sharing family life, he had the support he needed to die on his own terms, among his friends.

As great as Tom and his friends' achievements were, the institution trap ensnared him to the end. In this volume, it is for Benedikt Bjarnason, his mother Dóra and his friends (Chapter 22) – members of the first inclusion generation of twenty-somethings and their families – to discover how to align assistance so that people with substantial disabilities get to stretch the limits of interdependent community life without having first to fight their way out of the institution trap.

In 2001 Benedikt moved into his Reykjavík apartment and a bit later into part-time volunteer work with visitors at a nearby church. After Benedikt's inclusive schooling and attendance at a residential college in Denmark with a friend and classmate who also acted as his assistant, his mother saw this move as a logical next step in life as an active member of a society committed by policy to include people with substantial disabilities. Dóra negotiated government support for Benedikt to be at the centre of a demonstration project – Home with Support – designed to exemplify ways to realize Iceland's goal of a regular community life for people with disabilities. This demonstration project funds the assistance Benedikt needs to live in his own apartment and pursue a personalized schedule at about the same cost as he would incur by moving into a small group home and enrolling in a day service.

Benedikt benefits from a wide network of people, many of whom he is linked to through his family and a growing number of whom have come to know him in his own right. The design of his personal assistance system – which includes a board of directors dedicated to governing his personal services, a personal agent who co-ordinates his activities and assistances and paid assistants of about his own age – is adapted for Icelandic reality from approaches invented by North American families. In generating specific plans for Benedikt, Dóra has consulted professional friends and colleagues as well as young people who have known him through their school years together, sometimes playing a game of 'What would Benedikt say if he could talk?'. Dóra remains a powerful and important presence in his life even as she looks for ways to make space for his own friendships, interests and work. Rather than Benedikt losing legal standing by being subject to guardianship, his mother holds a power of attorney that authorizes her as his substitute decision-maker.

Like any important investigation, Benedikt's design for living trades room to learn for certainty. There are already plenty of questions to guide further learning: at what point might it be desirable to have a more stable group of assistants and how could this be achieved? Does more time at work make sense? How about work for pay? Are there ways to increase Benedikt's ability to communicate even further? How can the personal supports from friends and other committed people be sustained and strengthened even more? How would Benedikt's assistance be affected if his mother were less able to invest herself? What parts of Benedikt's assistance system can be adapted by other people and their families? What are the implications of Benedikt's discoveries for the way services are designed, funded and delivered?

So far it has been possible to pursue these important questions about interdependent living outside the net of the institution trap.

An agenda for moving on from institutionalization

To move on beyond institutions, people with disabilities and their families and allies of all ages and sorts of need for assistance need to mobilize public investment in flexible, individualized funding so that they can join Benedikt in making progress on this agenda:

- How do we move beyond treating isolated individuals toward support for important relationships?
- How do we move beyond casting people with intellectual disabilities and their families in passive roles – patient, client or consumer of service – toward alliances based on recognizing people's capacities to shape their own lives and co-produce necessary supports?
- How do we move beyond focusing action on professionally defined deficiencies toward building individualized capabilities through personalized and precise adaptations and assistance?

Making progress on these questions will take the courage and creativity to be inventive throughout a person's life. Regular practise of the strategies that Tom Allen used to fight off the worst effects of institutions will still be necessary. In particular, it will be important for people to reach out and gather more and more people into their lives, to find positive ways to make a contribution to their community's good, to stay in charge of their own story by telling and retelling it and to hold their dreams of freedom close.

Acknowledgements

I am grateful to Sean O'Brien for conversations on the strategies used by Irish Republican prisoners to resist the regime of nineteenth-century British prisons. These were helpful in framing Tom Allen's experiences in resisting twentieth-century institutions.

This chapter was written with funding to Responsive Systems Associates, Inc. from the National Institute on Disability and Rehabilitation, US Department of Education awarded to University of Minnesota under Grant Number H133B031116, CFDA #84.133 and a subcontract with Syracuse University. The opinions expressed herein are those of the authors, and no endorsement by the US Department of Education, the University of Minnesota or Syracuse University should be inferred.

References

Cambridge, P. (1999) 'Building care management competence in services for people with learning disabilities.' *British Journal of Social Work 29*, 393–415.

Lovett, H. (1996) *Learning to Listen: Positive Approaches and People with Difficult Behavior.* Baltimore, MD: Paul Brookes.

Nussbaum, M.C. (2004) *Hiding from Humanity: Disgust, Shame, and the Law.* Princeton, NJ: Princeton University Press.

O'Brien, J., Carssow, K., Jones, M., Mercer, M., Reynolds, L. and Strzok, D. (2003) *Never Give Up: Assets, Inc.'s Commitment to Community Life for People Seen as 'Difficult to Serve'.* Syracuse, NY: The Center on Human Policy, Syracuse University.

Traustadóttir, R. (1991) *Supports for Community Living.* Syracuse, NY: The Center on Human Policy, Syracuse University.

Vickers, G. (1970) *Freedom in a Rocking Boat: Changing Values in an Unstable Society.* London: Penguin.

Williams, R. (2004) *In a Struggling Voice: Selected Poems.* Philadelphia, MD: Temple University Institute on Disabilities.

Epilogue to Thomas F. Allen's Life Story

Rannveig Traustadóttir and Lisa Spina, USA

Tom died in March 1991 at the age of 78. He died at home in the apartment. His sister Marion was with him. Tom was buried in the family plot in Canisteo, his old home town. Before he died, Tom worked very hard on his story. As he grew weaker he realized he would not be able to finish it and asked Rannveig and Lisa to finish the story for him. Tom began writing his story many, many years ago when he was still living in the institution. In the beginning he wrote it to have something to do. As the years went by his attitude towards it changed, and he felt more and more compelled to tell the story of his life. He began to see his life story as his only chance to leave something behind. He also knew he was one of a small group of people who had managed to tell the story of life in the institution. His story could therefore be a testimony for so many others who were never heard. Over the years, many people have helped Tom write his story. Unfortunately, we only know who some of them are but we know that Tom wanted to thank all of them for their help. Tom was our friend. We loved him and we miss him.

Tom died peacefully in his sleep on 9 March 1991 at the age of 78. He died in his bed in the apartment. In the days before he died many people came to the apartment to say goodbye to him. His sister Marion, his only sibling left alive, was with him when he passed away. His brother Neal had died the year before. Tom had full consciousness and was fully coherent until he died.

Tom left instructions about his funeral. With Lisa's help he had made arrangements with a funeral home for the service and had paid for his burial and other funeral costs. According to his wishes he was buried in the family plot in Canisteo, his old home town. His nephew, who is a minister, performed the service. The funeral was on 12 March and the people attending were mostly his family. A few of his friends from Syracuse were there, mostly residents and staff from the apartment and other programmes run by the agency. Tom's friends in Syracuse held a memorial service for him in Syracuse on 18 March which was attended by a large group of people.

Tom worked very hard on his story the year before he died. As he grew weaker he realized he would not be able to finish it and asked the two of us to finish it for him. To make sure we had full authority to do so, he asked his lawyer to prepare a statement declaring that he wanted Rannveig Traustadóttir and Lisa Spina to finish his story. The statement also said that, if there were any royalties from his story, these should go to his family.

Tom began working on his story long before he met the two of us. He began writing his autobiography in the 1970s when he was at Craig Developmental Center. In the beginning he wrote it to have something to do. As the years went by his attitude towards the story changed and he felt more and more compelled to tell the story of his life. The feeling that his life had been wasted grew stronger and he began to see his life story as his only chance to leave something behind. He also realized that he was one of a very small group of people that lived in institutions who had managed to tell their story. His story could therefore be a testimony for so many others who were never heard.

It took an enormous amount of effort for Tom to tell his story. He had limited use of his arm and could not write the story himself so he had to dictate the story to other people who wrote it down for him. Tom had difficulties with his speech. It took a great deal of effort for him to speak and he spoke very slowly. He could only say a couple of words at a time and his words were hard to understand. Dictating his story to other people was therefore a very, very slow process which required a lot of patience for both Tom and the people helping him. Little by little, over a period of four years, Tom pieced the first part of his story together while living at Craig.

This first part of the story was about 25 typed pages which Tom called 'My Autobiography: A First Rough Draft'. It covered his childhood and his years at Rome and Craig. As far as we know, three people who worked in Craig and became his friends helped him with this first part of the story. While living at Syracuse Developmental Center (SDC), Tom added a few pages with the assistance of a staff member. After that he stopped writing for a while but started again after he had lived in the apartment for some time. It was mostly Lisa, but also some of the other staff at the apartment, who assisted him. When he died he left a pile of handwritten notes in addition to the first typed draft.

In his story, Tom does not name any of the people who helped him write it. We are not sure why but we suspect he wanted to avoid naming staff members who had become his friends. It was a bit of a risk for staff in the institution to become close friends with residents in those years. The administration did not like it. These people, who became his friends, not only assisted him to write his story, they also helped him survive the institution. Some of these people were instrumental in helping Tom move out of Craig and later out of SDC. Without this friendship and support Tom would not have been able to move out of the institution nor write his story. Unfortunately, we do not know the names of all the people who assisted Tom but we do know that he wanted to express his gratitude to everyone who supported him, cared for him and loved him. The people Tom wanted most of all to thank were his family, especially his brother Neal and his sister Marion. The person in his family he had the deepest love and respect for was his mother. He often told us that she was the most important person in his life. Without her he would not have had the happiest years of his life at home with his family as a child.

Other people Tom wanted to thank are Rosemary Burt, Carol Hayes Collier, Gail Donaldson, Darcy Miller Elks, Martin Elks, Sally Johnson, Michael Kennedy, Nidia Lopez, Marcus McKee, Sandy Nieciecki, Eric Paicoff, Christina Pezzulo, Angela Tarnacki, Linda Priest, Walter Priest, Gerry Womack, and all the other people who must remain anonymous because we do not know their names. Thank you all.

Tom's story is quite 'polite'. It is not written in an angry voice. He specifically told us that he did not want to sound bitter nor did he want to blame anyone. He knew it had been difficult for his family to send him to the institution and that his family felt guilty. He did not want to add to their pain. He therefore held back many of the worst things that happened to him and toned down the bad things he did talk about. His story is restrained. He certainly does not exaggerate.

Another issue which may have contributed to how politely Tom talks about his life in the institution is the fact that he was still living there when he was writing the first parts of the story and it could have been dangerous for him to write openly about the institutional horrors. There is no privacy in the institution and if someone had found his story, read it and reported him to the administration, it might have created great difficulties, for both himself and the friends who were helping him.

The story itself explains how Lisa came into Tom's life. She first met him when she started working in the apartment and later worked as his personal assistant. Through working with Tom, Lisa became his close friend. The first time Rannveig met Tom was in March of 1989. She was working on a large qualitative study, called 'The Community Study', which examined how people with intellectual disabilities were coping in the community, with a particular focus on social networks and personal relationships. Rannveig approached Tom and asked him if she could spend time with him and talk to him about his life and experiences. She thought it would be interesting to learn how a person who spent so many years in the institution, could – or could not – become a part of community life. Tom and Lisa welcomed her into their lives and she spent the next two years with them. What started as a research project developed into a close friendship.

Besides assisting in writing Tom's story, Rannveig has, with Tom and Lisa's permission, written a monograph describing some of Tom's experiences of institutions and the community and an analysis of the supports Lisa provided him with to enable him to reconnect with his family and the community (Traustadóttir 1991). Tom wanted his life to have a meaning and not be wasted and lost behind the walls of the institution. Like most of us, he wanted to leave something behind, to make a contribution, to be remembered. In honouring his wishes, Rannveig has given numerous talks about Tom's life, holding his story up as the contribution and lesson Tom wanted it to be. Part of the story is a photographic essay, making his story accessible to audiences who might have difficulties understanding long talks.

The two of us had very different roles in assisting Tom write his story. While Tom was still alive, Lisa worked with him on writing down the last part of the story. He also had long discussions with her about how he wanted his story to sound. He made it very clear he did not want to be negative or bitter. He trusted Lisa to make sure the story would have the right 'tone'.

Rannveig's role was to type up the different parts of the story and edit the many parts and versions into a coherent narrative. The first part of the story had been typed on a manual typewriter in the 1970s, and when Tom gave it to

Rannveig in 1989 it was about 15 years old and the print was beginning to fade. Rannveig retyped this part on to a computer before Tom died. After Tom's death the two of us collected all the typed and handwritten pages. Sorting through Tom's papers Lisa found two versions of the first part. Besides the typed part we had already seen, there was a handwritten version which differed from the typed one in a few places and there were old handwritten notes with additional information. Everything Tom had dictated after he moved out of Craig was handwritten. Rannveig took all this material and in the process of typing all these notes she became intimately familiar with Tom's way of telling his story which helped her do the editing job.

In editing his text we have had to make some decisions about which version of Tom's notes to use and what to leave out. In doing this we have relied on our knowledge of him and his wishes, as we knew them best. Although we have polished the text in some places we have tried to stay as true to his wording as possible. In describing himself and other disabled people Tom uses words that were common at the time. These are words such as 'cripple' and 'patient'. Although these may sound offensive to people today, we have kept these words to stay true to the historical accuracy of the text.

In his story, Tom does not say much about his disability. But he did talk about it with us and we want to share with you how he thought about his disability. We also want to document how his disability was defined at different times in the institutional records.

Although he had been so labelled, Tom never thought of himself as having an intellectual impairment. He saw himself as being physically impaired or 'crippled' as he called it in his story. Tom had very limited use of his arms. He never walked but could move his feet a little and could move himself around in a wheelchair by using his feet. His speech was hard to understand. Tom, however, never used any kind of communication aid. He wanted people to listen carefully and try to understand him. He did not mind repeating as often as it took for people to understand what he said. At first, people found him hard to understand but when they got used to his way of speaking it became much easier.

The institutional records describe him in different ways at different times. When Tom was readmitted to Rome State School in 1928 his records say:

> Has had infantile paralysis, chicken pox, measles, and whooping cough. Has never attended school. Boy is a cripple, cannot wait on himself... Has to be carried from place to place... Diagnosis: Imbecile. Mental exam: counted backward 20 to 1. IQ 37.

When Tom entered Craig Developmental Center in 1973 his records describe him as having 'borderline mental retardation' and in 1979 his records say he is 'non-mentally retarded'.

Both of us felt very close to Tom and considered him a dear friend. We have tremendous respect for how he managed to survive unspeakable difficulties in the institution – neglect, abuse, humiliation, isolation, abandonment and despair – and not be destroyed. He came out of the institution with faith in the goodness of other human beings and a willingness to trust them. He kept his dignity and was warm, gentle, caring, friendly and loving. He had a great sense of humour. He was very easy to like and love. It is difficult to describe Tom without sounding sentimental but the fact is that we consider ourselves privileged and proud to have known him. He was a truly remarkable human being.

Reference

Traustadóttir, R. (1991) *Supports for Community Living.* Syracuse, NY: Center on Human Policy, Syracuse University.

Contributors

Thomas F. Allen was born in 1912 in Canisteo, a small town in the state of New York in the United States. He was the second youngest of seven siblings. Tom was first institutionalized when he was about three years old but returned home at the age of six and spent a few happy years with his large and lively family. After his mother's death, he was institutionalized again when he was 15 years old and lived in three different state institutions for over 60 years. Tom did not want to die in the institution and fought a long battle to be released. Tom finally moved to the community in 1985 at the age of 72.

Christine Bigby is a senior lecturer and Director of Undergraduate Programs in the School of Social Work and Social Policy at LaTrobe University, Melbourne, Australia. She has been researching and teaching about intellectual disability for the past 16 years. Her particular interests have been in government policy, ageing with a lifelong disability and case management. She has published in both national and international journals and is author of two books: *Moving on Without Parents*, published by Elsevier Press (2000), and *Ageing with a Lifelong Disability: Policy, Program and Practice Issues for Professionals*, published by Jessica Kingsley Publishers (2004).

Dóra S. Bjarnason is a professor of sociology and disability studies at the Iceland University of Education. Her research focuses on inclusive education, disability studies, youth, social policy and equity. She has published widely both nationally and internationally and has authored two books in English: *School Inclusion in Iceland: The Cloak of Invisibility* (2003) and *Disability and Young Adulthood: New Voices from Iceland* (2004).

Paul Cambridge is a senior lecturer at the Tizard Centre at the University of Kent, England, teaching on a range of programmes and working directly with services and service users. His research interests include the long-term outcomes and costs of care in the community, deinstitutionalization, sexuality and HIV risk management, intimate and personal care, gender and caring roles and Queer theory. He is involved in EU-funded projects including anti-discrimination and intellectual disability projects. He has also produced a wide range of educational and staff training materials in intellectual disability, and currently edits the *Tizard Learning Disability Review*.

Jen Devers' awareness of disability issues is a lifelong interest, beginning with the life she shared growing up with her sister, Vicki, in a rural town in Victoria, Australia in the mid-1950s. When Vicki moved to Caloola, an institution for people with intellectual disabilities, Jen completed the Advanced Certificate in Community and Residential Studies (Disability Stream). She then started a programme named 'Leisure Friends' which aimed to reduce friendlessness and loneliness for people with a disability. She went on to teach students in disability studies. Jen has been involved in advocacy and service-delivery management for more than ten years. The influence of Vicki in her life has left her with an unshakeable belief in social justice and the need for inclusive communities for people with a disability.

Ian Freckelton is a barrister in full-time private practice in Melbourne, Australia. By night, he holds professorial positions in the Law Faculty and the Department of Psychological Medicine, as well as being an honorary associate professor in the Department of Forensic Medicine at Monash University. He holds a number of honorary positions at both Australian and overseas universities. In addition to editing a number of refereed journals which cross disciplinary boundaries, Ian is the author and editor of some two dozen books on health law, compensation law, criminal law, evidence law, coronial law, causation, policing and involuntary detention.

Julian Gardner is the Public Advocate in Victoria, Australia. This is a statutory office that has responsibility for the promotion and protection of the rights and interests of people with a disability. The Public Advocate acts as the guardian of last resort for people whose disability affects their capacity to make decisions about their accommodation, health care and other lifestyle matters. Julian has been a lawyer for over 30 years and held a number of public positions involving the rights of people who encounter various forms of disadvantage.

Ingiborg Eide Geirsdóttir lives in Reykjavík, Iceland. She spent more than 20 years in an institution but now lives on her own in an apartment in the community. Ingiborg has worked in the laundry of a large hospital in Reykjavík for many years. She writes poems and likes to walk and be out in nature.

Louise Glanville is the Senior Legal Adviser to the Attorney-General for the state of Victoria, Australia. Prior to taking on this role, Louise worked closely with Julian Gardner as the legal officer at the Office of the Public Advocate. Louise is trained in both law and social policy. She believes that the intersection of these two disciplines provides fruitful ground for considering human rights and the responses of the State to such rights.

Victor Hall spent his life until the age of 40 in institutions for people labelled as having an intellectual disability. Since then he has been living independently in the community in a council flat in Norwich, England, and has just retired after 20 years in the same job. He has a busy and active life in Norwich.

Avis Hunter spent the first 56 years of her life in institutions and temporary foster arrangements in different parts of the South Island of New Zealand. Since moving out of her 'last' institution in 1992, she has been committed to developing an increased understanding of her own life and to having some long-held questions answered. In 1995 she began working on her life story which was published in 1997. Avis's book, entitled *My Life*, was widely read and raised a great deal of awareness about the experience of institutionalization in her local community. The book was also adopted by a New Zealand playwright to provide the basis of an experimental play which was performed in Dunedin in 1998.

Emil Johansen is the pseudonym of a man who lives in a small community in northern Norway. He has physical and cognitive impairments, and grew up in a segregated institution where he received little help. He has been living in his own home in the community for the past decade, spending time with his girlfriend and some new friends who live nearby, and especially enjoying his favourite hobby of fishing.

Kelley Johnson is a senior lecturer in the School of Social Science and Planning at RMIT University in Melbourne, Australia. She has worked as a researcher and advocate with people with intellectual disabilities for 15 years and has published widely on deinstitutionalization, women's issues and inclusion. Her latest book, co-authored with Jan Walmsley, is *Inclusive Research with People with Learning Disabilities: Past, Present and Futures*, published by Jessica Kingsley Publishers (2003).

Kristjana Kristiansen is Associate Professor in the Department of Social Work and Health Sciences at the Norwegian University of Science and Technology (NTNU) in Trondheim, Norway, where she teaches research methods, gender studies and disability studies at postgraduate level. Her educational background is in psychology and public health, and her current research interests are in the field of mental health, living conditions for marginalized groups, violence and abuse, and inclusive research methodology and a lived-experience approach. She has 30 years' experience working in various human-service fields, as an advocate, service provider, teacher and researcher, and has published numerous books and articles.

Brigit Mirfin-Veitch is Avis Hunter's friend and writing partner. Brigit and Avis have known each other for seven years and work together on writing projects of mutual interest. Brigit is also a qualitative researcher with the Donald Beasley Institute, a national institute which conducts research and education in the area of intellectual disability in New Zealand.

John O'Brien learns about building more just and inclusive communities from people with disabilities, their families and their allies. He uses what he learns to advise people with disabilities and their families, advocacy groups, service providers and governments, and to spread the news among people interested in change by writing and through workshops. He is affiliated with the Center on Human Policy (USA), the Northwest Training and Development Team (UK), and the Marsha Forest Centre: Inclusion. Family. Community (Canada).

Patricia O'Brien is a dean in the Faculty of Postgraduate Studies and Research, Auckland College of Education, New Zealand. Within the faculty Patricia teaches several modules at the Master's level in disability studies. Her research interests and publications include deinstitutionalization, advocacy and inclusive education.

Sheena Rolph worked for 12 years in adult education for people with intellectual disabilities who were living in a large hospital outside Norwich, England. She then undertook oral history and archival research for her PhD thesis, 'The History of Community Care for People with Learning Difficulties in Norwich, 1930–1980: The Role of Two Hostels'. She is a research fellow at the UK's Open University, continuing to work on her chosen field of the social history of community care for people with intellectual disabilities.

Lisa M. Spina has a degree in special education. She has worked with people with intellectual disabilities as an advocate, direct-care worker and administrator for many years. Lisa was Tom Allen's friend and his personal assistant during the last years of his life. Lisa is currently the Assistant Program Coordinator of Self Directed Personal Services for United Cerebral Palsy in Syracuse, New York, USA.

Gudrún V. Stefánsdóttir is Assistant Professor at the Iceland University of Education and a doctoral student at the University of Iceland. Her thesis is based on life histories of people with intellectual disabilities born 1924–1950. She has worked with people with intellectual disabilities for many years as an advocate, care worker and lately as a researcher.

Steven J. Taylor is Director of the Center on Human Policy, Coordinator of Disability Studies and Professor of Education at Syracuse University. He also serves as editor of *Mental Retardation*, an interdisciplinary journal published by the American Association on Mental Retardation (AAMR). He has published widely on the sociology of disability, inclusion, disability policy and qualitative research methods. He was the recipient of AAMR's 1997 Research Award and received the Syracuse University Chancellor's Citation for Exceptional Academic Achievement in 2003.

Ethel Mary Temby formerly worked as a teacher at primary and secondary level and later in adult literacy with the Council of Adult Education, Victoria, Australia. Ethel has six children of whom Rowan is the youngest. After his birth she became active in trying to improve many unjust situations experienced by families with intellectually disabled children. She became a strong advocate for human and citizen rights, and for the closing of institutions, with community living and appropriate support replacing them. The award of a Churchill Fellowship in 1976 led to her study of best practices in all aspects of living for people with intellectual disabilities. The study was carried out in the UK, Sweden, the USA and Canada. Much of this influenced Victorian legislation. Ethel served on Ministerial Advisory Committees and was closely involved in Citizen Advocacy development, Parent to Parent support and other initiatives.

Magnus Tideman has a PhD in social work, and is Senior Lecturer, concentrating on disability studies, at Halmstad University in Sweden. His research has focused on living conditions for people with disabilities and questions about 'normality' and 'deviance' in schools. He is series editor (with Ove Mallander) of an English-speaking series on Nordic disability research entitled *Social Research on Disability*, published by Studentlitteratur, Lund, Sweden.

Jan Tøssebro is Professor of Social Work at the Norwegian University of Science and Technology (NTNU), Trondheim, Norway. For 15 years Jan was involved in evaluation and follow-up studies of the Norwegian deinstitutionalization reform. He has also been involved in research on school integration, children with disabilities and the study of disabled peoples' living conditions. Jan currently chairs the Norwegian State Council on Disability and is a member of a committee appointed to propose new/revised disability legislation. He has three children, including a young man with autism and an intellectual disability.

Rannveig Traustadóttir is Professor in the Faculty of Social Science at the University of Iceland in Reykjavík. She has worked with people with disabilities as an advocate, direct-support worker, administrator, policy-maker and researcher since the late 1960s. Rannveig received her doctoral training at Syracuse University in the USA between 1986 and 1992. During that time she met Tom Allen and became involved in assisting him write his story. Rannveig has published widely in the area of disability. She has been active in Nordic disability research and is currently the president of NNDR, the Nordic Network on Disability Research.

Jan Walmsley is currently Assistant Director at the Health Foundation in London and is Visiting Professor in the History of Learning Disability at the Open University, UK. She has been interested in the history of learning disability since the mid-1980s, and has written extensively in this area. She is currently working on a history of community care for people with learning disabilities entitled *Care, Control and Citizenship*, to be published by Palgrave in 2006.

Subject Index

Author Index